YOGA
for the
WOUNDED HEART

A Journey, Philosophy, and Practice
of Healing Emotional Pain

TATIANA FORERO PUERTA

Lantern Books ● New York

2018
Lantern Books
128 Second Place
Brooklyn, NY 11231
www.lanternbooks.com

Some names and identifying details of people and places in this book have been changed to protect the privacy of individuals.

Printed in the United States of America

Library of Congress Cataloging-in-Publication Data

Names: Puerta, Tatiana Forero, author.
Title: Yoga for the wounded heart : a journey, philosophy, and practice of healing emotional pain / Tatiana Forero Puerta.
Description: Brooklyn : Lantern Books, 2018. | Includes bibliographical references.
Identifiers: LCCN 2017058214 (print) | LCCN 2018003380 (ebook) | ISBN 9781590565797 (ebook) | ISBN 9781590565780 (pbk.)
Subjects: LCSH: Yoga. | Healing. | Pain.
Classification: LCC B132.Y6 (ebook) | LCC B132.Y6 P84 2018 (print) | DDC 204/.36—dc23
LC record available at https://lccn.loc.gov/2017058214

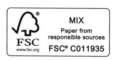

MIX
Paper from
responsible sources
FSC
www.fsc.org
FSC® C011935

To Vanne, who was there.
And for my parents, Jairo and Olga:
This wouldn't exist without you; this wouldn't exist with you.

Contents

Workbook: The Five Practices

Fundamentally, we understand all the highest things.
—Søren Kierkegaard

PART I

The Yoga of Yoga

1

THE BREAKDOWN AND
THE JOURNEY HOME

When I was twenty-two years old, I had a massive physical, emotional, mental, and spiritual breakdown. It was as though the years of accumulated trauma and stress I'd managed to keep under wraps could no longer be stifled. All of the secrets had been compacted and locked away deep inside myself, but whatever was there had tripled or quadrupled in size and morphed into what felt like a beast. It had suddenly become self-aware and was effectively breaking out of the chest I'd carved for it, the way someone presumed dead and mistakenly buried might kick and scream and claw their way out of their coffin—with urgency, might, and desperation. The scratching and pounding got louder, and my beast would no longer go unnoticed. I couldn't contain its density or intensity much longer, and sensed a countdown had begun.

I had moved by myself to New York City in an attempt to leave behind everything I'd known. I didn't know a soul, and that's what I thought I wanted. Perhaps the breakdown was due to the anonymity of the Big Apple, with its millions of nameless faces, or the city's continual movement—like a self-perpetuating pendulum. Maybe it was the sheer coldness of that autumn, or simply the fact that no matter how much you try, you simply can't run away from yourself, or from what you've hidden from yourself.

Maybe it was the perfect synchronization of these elements that produced that stark loneliness—the ideal breeding ground for the ghouls of my youth to arrive at my door. They knocked and knocked and eventually tore the door down. Before I knew it, I found myself descending into a massive vortex of depression, which showed up in a variety of costumes. That is to say, it manifested as a number of ailments more commonly recognizable as diagnoses: extreme panic disorder, post-traumatic stress disorder, obsessive compulsive disorder, anorexia, self-mutilation, and suicidal tendencies. They were all branches of the same tree of illness.

They say that you should write what you know, and Lord knows I've known madness as much as you can know just about anything in this life. I've known darkness powerful enough to confuse you out of your own identity and convince you that nothing matters. It sneaks in between the sheets with you at night, right before you doze off. It gets comfy and whispers unmentionables. It finds you on the train. It sits next to you while you're trying to work, impatiently tapping its fingers. It becomes ubiquitous, like the sound of traffic you no longer hear as separate from life itself.

This darkness convinces you that life is worth nothing, and not in the bohemian and sexy Sartrean sense where you're inspired to write, paint, and create masterpieces based on the absurdity of life's inherent meaninglessness. It evangelizes nihilism, but not the type where you sit at a café chain-smoking Gauloises, eating imported cheeses, sipping on French wine, and toasting Camus and Nietzsche. Nope. This darkness has you scouring your life for a reason to exist and somehow you find nothing. Your morning prayer consists of asking that God finally run you over with a bus. You spend days not moving, because it's all too painful and your bones feel as heavy as anvils, and the thought of sinking to the core of the planet sounds like respite, so *good*.

Yet, I also know healing quite well. In fact, each day that passes I know healing better than I know meaninglessness. I can attest to that fact because I'm here, writing this book, living my life, and I can't remember the last time I truly wished I were dead. I know healing, and I know how much effort and courage it requires: the staggering level of commitment and the mind-boggling amount of faith. I also know how worth it it all was, and still is—and that is why I am writing. The fruit of that harvest is just *that* sweet, and so, so worth it. The lessons from the journey of healing are unique for each one of us and simultaneously a basic part of what it means to be human, what it means to abide in this world: together.

I've always been deeply fascinated by the fact that every major religious and spiritual tradition addresses the question of suffering—that is, why do we suffer? Suffering is an inescapably human condition, as integral to our experience as breathing. For me, this is enough of a reason to dive into it, explore it, and see what it has to say. In a deeply wounded world full of suffering, I believe that with enough work and concerted effort it is not only possible but imperative for us to heal our own personal hurt, not only so *we* can heal, but for the enrichment and growth of our families, our communities, and our world. It behooves us to take on the healing journey, for we cannot have a healthy, healed world if we are not doing our own work toward our own health in heart and mind.

Ram Dass once said that we are all just walking each other home, and I couldn't agree more. However, we stand at a time and in a culture that have somehow managed to forget the rites of passage that were once a vital part of our human ancestry and of the history of our consciousness as a species. These rituals, practiced for thousands of years, exposed us to the elements of life and nature and transitioned us out of childhood with respect for and an experiential understanding of natural laws. No longer is it normative to learn to connect to the flow of life itself, to nurture our relationship with the most foundational aspects of our existence: change, fear, and death. Far too often in our modern world, we go about life blindly, with no way to know in which direction the winds are blowing or what that might mean for our crops, the hunt, our tribe (meaning now our work, our families, our communities), or even the minutiae of our daily endeavors.

In our history as a species, we have developed astonishing technologies, advanced scientifically in myriad and unimaginable ways, and achieved feats of medicine never thought possible. Perhaps we have also diverged from our most primordial and pervasive center: our own hearts. We have, in many ways, lost our way home. The heart—our center—is our place of intuition, compassion, and recognition of where we stand in our relationship to life, our environment, and one another. Our lives have grown exponentially chaotic and disconnected, and in this state, we suffer.

Any exploration of suffering is an exploration of our misdirection, of the circumstances and choices that have taken us away from our hearts, our inner guidance system; that have separated us from who we truly are. The magic lies here: In the work of exploring our lost-ness, we find the journey home—to connection, awareness, and laughter; to enjoying the breeze on an autumn day; to becoming wholly immersed in the melody of a song; to conversations, holding hands, hugs, playfulness, joy, and harmony; to the center from which all these things effortlessly flow. Love.

As I have said in many of my classes, there was my life before yoga, and my life after the conscious decision to become a devoted student of this rich and ancient lineage— my decision to *practice* yoga. That's why I intend to share with you my story, as well as the tools and teachings that guided me out of the darkness of suffering. I don't do this because I think my story is special or unique. The opposite is in fact the case. I share it because it's a story like all our stories. All of us have lost our path in one way or another; all of us have faced fear and death; all of us have in one moment or another desperately sought to come home. The practice of yoga for me has been a thread left by the wise and ancient to guide me out of the labyrinth. It has also been a boot camp. It has worked me to the bone and required me to face truly difficult things. In so doing, it has been my medicine, and it has mended me.

Yoga is a growing phenomenon in the West, one that will continue to expand as people settle into its many teachings and reap its undeniable benefits. But the philosophy and wisdom of its teachings often take a back seat to the physical practice. For this reason, I hope within these pages to shed some light on—or rather, to bring to life—some of the most fundamental yet powerful teachings and principles of the practice of yoga.

With tears in his eyes, a great teacher of mine once pleaded with us, his students, never to allow yoga to be only about the physical postures. He said that way was akin to riding a unicycle instead of in a limousine: the practice of movement was but one small piece of what yoga had to offer its practitioners; its philosophy was the larger vehicle. What if we climbed in and went for a ride? What if we embraced this amazing practice as a highly developed technology of consciousness rather than prescriptive dogma? What if we allowed it to unfold before us as light on the path and a guide on the journey, and then, as the journey itself? For it's here, in the treacherous and won-drous middle of the path, that the heart blooms and truly heals. It's here, right where we stand, that we begin our journey home.

2

THERE MUST BE SOMETHING MORE

THE KEY TO THE MAP OF BEING-NESS

Yoga, above all, is an experiential practice; it's about what works, what is useful. The philosophical and psychological underpinnings as provided by the yogic sages' ancient writings simply give us a container—language and concepts that help us hold and mediate this wondrous experience of being alive. Because, let's face it, who at some point has not felt utterly lost?

When on the fifteenth anniversary of my father's death I attempted to take my own life, I made contact with a part of the abyss that is available to human consciousness. The encounter involved a loss of meaning so profound that the pain resulting from it felt worse than the possibility of no longer being around to experience anything at all. I was—or, more accurately, I *experienced* myself to be—entirely isolated as I sat in my small room in Brooklyn, holding a razor blade in one hand and staring at the open bottles of antidepressants, painkillers, and muscle relaxers on my bedside table.

* * *

The yogic sages were concerned with experience and ontology—the study of being and the experience of self. The writers of these mystical and yet, as we will soon explore, pragmatic texts suggest that it is unfortunate that we take *being* for granted. Because we can't *not* be, we don't take time to truly inquire as to the nature of being-ness. Instead, we go on about our daily business most often enmeshed in a cycle—one task, place, project, job, or relationship to the next—until there comes, maybe suddenly or gradually, a perhaps unavoidable existential anxiety. This anxiety will throw us into the questions, Who am I? What am I doing with my life? and Does any of this matter?

Often, these questions are precipitated by huge shifts in our circumstances—loss of a job, divorce, death, or another form of suffering—and all of a sudden, we hit a wall. We realize we've been living blindly, or perhaps not living at all. Our life feels fake. The ancient teachers of yoga would agree: yup, our lives are a farce. All of it is an illusion. Yet we know that feeling of *There must be something more.* Well, that's completely right on—and *that*, that *right-on-ness*, is precisely the inquiry at hand. What is *that*? How do we get there and ditch the illusion? What's the point of all of it?

To the philosophical skeptic and the pragmatist, the following questions might arise: To what degree is coming to a conclusion on the nature of my "being-ness" going to help me get ahead in my day-to-day life? How is pondering the meaning of existence valuable in a world that runs at speeds so great that technological advances are rendered outdated in only a couple years? Isn't it just navel-gazing? And even if it isn't, what's the point if philosophy can offer no answers but only raise more questions?

To that, I say: Yoga is a healing art. The philosophy of yoga is medicine. We can only ever truly speak from our own experience, and from that place I can bear witness. Yoga took the blade out of my hand and the pills off my shelf. It put my mind at peace, a smile on my face, and the meaning of my life back in my hands. *Yoga saved my life.*

Although I use my own story throughout these pages to explore the way this philosophy—this *practice*—has transformed me, the anecdotes are examples, not "proof." So, what *is* the proof? *Ehipassiko.* This original Pali phrase translates to "come and see for yourself"; the ultimate proof is your own experience, not mine. In fact, all sound science rests on the principle of replicability. What I ask the skeptic is this: Why not engage in this as a sort of experiment? In the end, what do you have to lose?

As for the sages responsible for the philosophy, it might be reassuring to know that they weren't interested in navel-gazing, either. They were concerned with what's useful just as much as we are. In fact, as Sri Swami Satchidananda—a venerated teacher of these texts—points out, modern science is essential. Scientists can gain useful information about anything, from the behavior of electrons to how dolphins communicate, and through study and analysis make valuable predictions that help us understand and mediate the natural world. The primary tool of the scientist—that which she cannot go without and integral to her hypotheses and discoveries—is the same primary tool of yoga: observation.

The difference is the object being observed. The natural scientist observes the external world; the yogi the internal landscape. The philosophy and psychology of yoga, then, is a map through the often-uncharted territory of our own awareness. The primary principles of yoga as found in the *Yoga Sūtras of Patañjali* are the key to that map; with them, we can enter into understanding of the one thing we can be sure of: our being-ness. For, as René Descartes famously noted, *Cogito ergo sum*—"I think, therefore I am": Our own consciousness is the most indubitable thing there is.

A Little Bit of Context

Before we dive in, it might be helpful to understand what the *Yoga Sūtras* are, or even what a *sūtra* is and how it pertains to our discussion at hand. Because I am neither a historian nor an anthropologist, I will provide an admittedly crude contextualization of the *Yoga Sūtras*.[1] To begin, the word *sūtra* stems from the Sanskrit *sutr*, which gives us our English word *suture*. To suture is to sew, and a *sūtra* is a metaphorical thread. One of my teachers once said to me that he liked to think of *sūtras* as strands of thread on which to place beads of wisdom that he could wear around his neck, close to his heart.

Sūtras are writings—short aphorisms that are simple to the eye and easy to recall (and in the original Sanskrit even more so, because a collection of *sūtras* often has a particular cadence, making them songlike and hence easier to memorize). The external simplicity of a *sūtra* (usually one or two sentences long) is misleading. Upon close inspection, it's easy to recognize that these pithy statements conceal layers upon layers of meaning—applicable, changeable, adaptable, and insightful no matter how many times we return to them.

The *Yoga Sūtras* are a collection of 196 short statements that concern the topic of yoga, divided into four parts: Contemplation, Practice, Accomplishments, and Absoluteness. Our discussion will revolve primarily around the first fifty-one *sūtras*, as they form the foundation for the rest of the work. The second portion (the following fifty-five *sūtras*) contains what is commonly referred to as the Eight Limbs of Yoga, which concerns the behavioral practices that one engages in (or avoids) on the yogic path. Although we will touch on some of these, the Eight Limbs are fairly accessible and applicable, and much more commentary can be found on them in contemporary literature on yoga.[2] The last two portions of the *sūtras* concern the subtler realms of consciousness available on the path of yoga. A discussion of these is beyond the scope of this book.

It is relevant to note that the study of the *Yoga Sūtras of Patañjali* is a practice all on its own. Even in the discussion at hand, I will not be laying out an explanation for each *sūtra*, and we won't cover every single *sūtra* in the first portion. In sum, this book is *not* meant to be an exhaustive explanation/translation of the *Yoga Sūtras*. Instead, it is intended to provide a primer for the most critical concepts that act as a foundation for change in our lives—in particular, for how we heal from suffering.

This begs the question, Why the *Yoga Sūtras*? The *Yoga Sūtras of Patañjali* is the first text that expounds on yoga as a system. Unlike many texts written and studied around the same era, the *Yoga Sūtras* is not story-based. Instead, it provides a clear structure specifically dealing with unraveling yoga proper. For this reason, the *Yoga Sūtras of Patañjali* has become the primary text of yoga philosophy in the modern age.

All of this may not seem particularly consequential, until you (a) experience the text itself, which we will get to following this brief contextualization; and (b) recognize that prior to its inception, the teachings presented in the *Sūtras* were not accessible to any but a lucky few. Now, I'll reiterate that I'm neither a trained historian nor an anthropologist, but I *am* a philosopher, and one thing philosophers are interested in is the development of ideas over time. One of the reasons for this interest is because tracing such changes can perhaps tell us something about the nature of shifts in human consciousness, concerns, and values.

Historically speaking, this past "knowledge" or "discussion" on yoga was very minimal. The word *yoga* appeared very sparingly in other ancient texts. The *Vedas* and *Upaniṣads* mention it in passing; and although the *Bhagavad Gītā*, the principal text of Hindu thought, does expound on different forms of yoga, it does so alongside other big ideas like dharma, family, and destiny. No other texts delve *exclusively* into the inner workings of yoga proper.

Additionally, the ancient texts were not meant to be read by just anyone. Leaving aside the limited literacy rate thousands of years ago (the *Sūtras* are dated between four and two thousand years BCE), these texts were meant to be studied alongside a teacher and were carried through a rich lineage of oral tradition before they were jotted down. Although a hint of that lineage remains in the *Sūtras* (almost every translation of the *Sūtras* you encounter today will be accompanied by commentary), the *Yoga Sūtras of Patañjali* was the first time in history that yoga was addressed in one place, at one time, in a clear, systematized fashion. In fact, the very first *sūtra*, the introduction to the whole thing, reads as follows (*drumroll, please*): "Now, the teachings of yoga."[3,4]

Who Cares about Yoga?

Fair enough, you may say. *But what is all this hoopla about yoga, anyway? So what if the*
Sūtras *are the first text that expounds on yoga. Why is yoga so special?*

Aha! And now, let *us* begin our journey. Why *is* yoga so special? The answer to
that question, and in fact the key to the very first *sūtra* itself, lies in the definition and
etymology of the word *yoga*. And so, let the yoga begin.

3
YOGA ISN'T YOGA

I'm going to break the news right off the bat: Yoga does not mean Downward-Facing Dog. Yoga also does not mean "Rock Star" pose, Lululemon butt-hugging pants, or designer yoga mats. Obviously, two to five thousand years ago, Patañjali had *zero* idea about any of these things, and yet the imagery that arises when we say the word *yoga* today is of neo-hippies with tight buns and overpriced gym clothes, legs twisted around their necks like pretzels.

Even for those of us who build our lives (diets, schedules, and routines) around our yoga practices, the word *yoga* doesn't even mean "conscious patterned movement and mindful breathing." Nor does it mean getting into a forearm stand without wrinkling your forehead. Nor does it mean expanding the body, mind, heart, and breath—all the nice sentiments we may hear (and which I'm guilty of uttering plenty of times) during yoga class. So, what *is* yoga?

The word *yoga* stems from the Sanskrit root *yuj*, which means to bind, yoke, harness, or bring together. In the context at hand, *yoga* is both a verb and a noun, simultaneously referring to both a thing you "do," a practice, and what I have come to call "the happy accident" that occurs *from* that practice. As a verb, the word connotes the continual activity of bringing something together. That begs the question, What is set apart? This is where the ontology—the study of existence, being, and becoming—begins.

The State of Separation

If you're human, you've at one point or another felt alone. You may have even felt the twinge of the existential moment, or even the unstoppable downward spiral of the existential crisis. The last of these was my form of acquaintance with the state of separation, which can manifest in different ways. In my case, it came with a slew of titles: depression, PTSD, OCD, SI (self-injury), and other conditions that served to classify me and my experience—my "problems." My late teens and early twenties were a smorgasbord of mental-health issues as colorful as all the pills I had to take on a daily basis—a serving of about twenty by the time I hit bottom.

It's an all-too-familiar story. Take the white pill so you can be in public without passing out from fear. But that's going to trigger migraines, so take the red one at any sign of flashing lights in your peripheral vision. But that might set off the heart palpitations, so this green and pink one will help. But because you might be prone to seizures, take this blue one to decrease that likelihood, and simply repeat three times a day. *That* was my daily reality. But what other option did I have, really? It wasn't as though my *body* wasn't showing alarming signs. (I lost count of the times I fainted in public or had to sit to catch my breath because it felt like my heart would spontaneously combust.) And when your body is sick, you do your due diligence: go to the doctor and take the medicine you're given you so you can get better. Right?

It was more than just the heart arrhythmia—those scary, uncomfortable palpitations—or losing consciousness at random intervals. What ailed me more than the physical symptoms was internal: I couldn't comprehend how people survived from one day to the next, how everyone seemed to be okay in such a wounded world. I didn't get that. I couldn't grasp how people managed to ride trains, meet new people, hang out at bars, and go about their day not paralyzed by fear of what might happen next—a train wreck. An earthquake. A terrorist attack. Was everyone completely unaware, I wondered, that at any moment they could just cease to be? That at any second the people they loved most could just die, and that would be . . . *it*? Was it not clear to everyone, as it was clear to me, that there are no holy moments; every minute is fair game for disaster? It often seemed to me that no one wanted to address the big fat elephant in the room of existence itself. Meanwhile, I couldn't keep my eyes off it.

I simply couldn't pretend. I've been the definition of "the sensitive person" since I can remember, the type whose nervous system seems to lie on top of the skin rather than underneath it. I was told from early on to grow thicker skin, to stop crying, to (in my mother's words) "harden up that little heart," or else life would be, well, really hard. Emotions plaster themselves on my face like gaudy makeup. Even when I'm trying to hide how I feel, my face always broadcasts the truth.

So, I was deeply afraid and there was no masking it. And being afraid of existence itself means being afraid of a host of other things: spiders, the dark, loneliness, crowds, elevators, heights, going to sleep, not sleeping enough, food, gaining weight, indigestion, migraine headaches, going crazy, losing it (really losing it!). Because all of it—every single one of these things I feared—led me down the same rabbit hole and straight into the arms of the one thing I feared most of all: death.

Philosopher Martin Heidegger said that one of our most basic existential traits is that we are being-toward-death. Death is the one thing from which we can't flee, and this is our existential situation—simply part of our inheritance from life. When we ignore the truth of our situation, says Heidegger, we're apt to lead inauthentic lives—lives unexamined and taken for granted. Lives like these, as Socrates said, are really not worth living.

My problem was never acknowledging that I was being-toward-death. It was quite the opposite, in fact. Death had taken it upon himself to chase me on a motorcycle, trying to whack me with his shiny sickle. I had a head start but he was gaining on me. At least, that's what it felt like. I wasn't in denial that I was going to die. I knew exactly where I stood in relationship to the game of existence. If anything, I was hyperaware of my existential situation and had looked into the face of death on more occasions than most people my age had.

By the age of fourteen, I'd witnessed the death of both of my parents, and some years later, that of my childhood best friend. By the time I was seventeen, I'd had a gun pointed at me twice. Before I could understand how fear operates, I'd already been immersed in its dark waters, my life, and everything that mattered to me, disintegrated before my eyes. Before my mind was able to comprehend what death even was, I'd already developed an acute intimacy with it. I'd felt firsthand the way that subtle and elusive *somethingness* that is life withdraws in a second, turning the once animate into a stillness so profound it cannot be named, although it can surely be sensed. And it scared me shitless.

Amid all the pain, sheer discomfort, and desire to run away, my day-to-day experience overflowed with morbid anxiety and disturbing night terrors by the time I hit my early twenties. As I slept, I'd have flashbacks of my parents' deaths, then be unable to look away. Often, I'd wake up sprawled over the bathtub, scissors in hand, trying to figure out how I managed to disassemble half the kitchen in my sleep yet again and why my pajama pants were all cut up. I'd return to my bed to find scissors and knives scattered on the floor around it. It was sheer madness: the make-believe mixed up with the real; waking life and dream-land merging into one another almost seamlessly.

I felt crazy. How do you explain to people that life feels raw, everything is scary, and you struggle to get through the day? How can you connect with others when you question your own sanity? The alienation grew in intensity my first year in New York City, as I was starting graduate work in, perhaps ironically, philosophy and comparative religion, fields that by their very nature are about the study of meaning itself. In the sea of people that I would encounter on the L train as I made my way from Bushwick in Brooklyn to New York University in Manhattan, I couldn't relate to a single person. Everyone seemed so calm to me, so unaffected. I envied strangers daily, so unmoved by all those little things they seemed to take for granted: getting into a crowded subway car, walking down the street, sanity, and even life itself. I couldn't take any of it for granted. None of these things felt simple to me.

In my bedroom at night I could overhear the person in the room adjacent to mine playing indie music records; witty little lyrics resonated through the apartment as though life was just peachy. Isolation descended on me like an impermeable San Francisco fog, and any flashlight I tried to shine in an attempt to pierce the skies and find my way out only intensified the glare, and blinded me further. Amid piles of papers, stacks of books, and my ephemeral diversions—a guitar, a pack of smokes, and a fresh stack of razor blades should it come to that—I was utterly separated. It wasn't just that I'd come to New York alone. It was something else. Something about this time and place brought everything to a boil inside of me and would not allow all the experiences of my tumultuous childhood to rest unexamined any longer.

I thought that I'd been living Socrates' examined life by devoting myself to the study of meaning itself. The truth was I'd fled to these doorways of theoretical meaning as a way to make sense of my own troubled childhood: of the pain, deaths, and deep sorrow. But in the end, my intellectual pursuits served as an escape from my day-to-day life, from where I stood and what I'd lived through. So long as I had my head buried in a book, I wouldn't have to think about my past, or my pain. Yet, I somehow thought that I'd managed to overcome my history, simply by giving it a cursory assessment, saying, *Yes, well, that's in the past. I'm over that now,* and instead depending on my fierce independence. Somehow, I'd convinced myself that I'd forgotten it all and it no longer affected me. Boy, was I wrong!

Coming to New York was like stepping into a haunted house of all my own ghosts, and like one of those freaky and clichéd movies, once I entered, all the doors closed behind me, locking me in. All of a sudden, it was as though I could hear the howls of my own unresting spirits, those things I thought I'd buried deep within. They were waking up. All the memories reappeared and came closer; they seemed to beckon louder, calling for a return to the most basic of all inquiries: *Who am I? Who am I?* I knew, though, that to answer this question I would have to face the specters of my past, and recall names, places, and occurrences so bitter and toxic that my mouth hadn't uttered them in almost a decade. Reestablishing who I was would mean unearthing memories so painful I had legitimately lost access to a good number of them, leaving only a false blankness in their place. I had to face the unfaceable. Overwhelmed by fear and loneliness, and utterly lost, I had no idea where to start. So, I chose an easier route. I looked at the razor blades on my nightstand and decided to end it all.

4

VISION AND VEILS

Imagine strolling into an optometrist without an appointment and putting on a random pair of prescription glasses. It's not your prescription; in fact, your eyesight is perfect. But you walk in anyhow and put on glasses that distort your vision so much that you trip walking out of the store and stumble onto the sidewalk. As you make your way down the street, you use your hands to feel your way around, to orient you. You look around and everything looks off; people's faces seem contorted and the sidewalk is twisted. You get to your car and sloppily drive away. Let's pretend you don't cause an accident, and you make it home. After some time, the new glasses start to feel okay, and you say to yourself, *I could get used to this.*

Humans are creatures of habit—we all know that—and we tend to adapt to circumstances fairly well. It's said that a year after a major catastrophe like losing a limb or a major positive change like winning the lottery, our basic state of happiness returns to a baseline: wherever we tended to be before these huge changes took place. So, as humans, we become accustomed to our surroundings and make do with what we have. It's then quite likely that after wearing these glasses for a while you won't want to take them off. And if someone made you, your regular vision would feel distorted.

We all wear glasses. Throughout our lives, we collect and adapt to different prescriptions, even different-colored lenses. Some we get from our parents or other role models; others we adopt from friends or people we surround ourselves with, the way we tend to pick up catchphrases or mannerisms from those closest to us. Sometimes, we place one pair of glasses over another and start a small collection on our heads— even if they don't match, and even if their effects counteract one another. Experiences that hurt us—deep childhood traumas in particular—can cause us to adopt a variety of especially strong lenses through which we then see our world.

We may use one pair of lenses because they help us understand things in our lives that might not make sense to us as we're experiencing them. A friend who was making a concerted effort to stop smoking once told me a story about how his son, five at the time, told his wife, "Don't worry, Mommy. Daddy put on the patch so if he tries to pick up a cigarette the patch will make him drop it." I thought it was both adorable and also quite accurate and insightful. In an attempt to understand the world, it's only natural that we create stories. Jack, my friend's son, will grow up and learn that even though his father was wearing a patch, there was still choice involved in his decision to quit smoking, and Jack's interpretation of that event will naturally change as he matures and his understanding develops.

Yet it's not always so easy to switch our lenses in light of new information. Sometimes, we may refuse to remove our interpretative lenses beyond the time they are useful. Perhaps as a second grader we were bitten by a big dog and adopted the lens that all big dogs are bad, and thus grew up with a fear and avoidance of big dogs. Then, say one day a big dog is in danger and we happen to be at the right place at the right time to save its life. If we are stuck with the old lens and its effects, we may not save the dog. The point is this: Lenses may wear out their usefulness and keep us from seeing things as they are. As a result, they influence the way we feel, our belief structures, and hence the decisions we make.

Our behavior is largely influenced by the lenses through which we interpret the events of our lives at any given moment. The problem arises in that much of the time we are ignorant of the fact that we're wearing any lenses at all. The *sutras* refer to this state of being as *avidyā*: wrong-seeing, non-seeing, misguided perception, or ignorance. *Avidyā* is one of the five obstacles (*kleśas*) from waking up out of suffering, and in fact, all obstacles that keep us in the throes of suffering stem from this unseeing.[5]

If *avidyā*, this state of non-apprehension, is at the root of our suffering, then what is it, exactly? In other words, what is it that we aren't seeing correctly that is responsible for our grief? The *Sūtras'* answer is fairly simple: We live in a state of ignorance when we confuse the impermanent as permanent, the painful as pleasant, and the self as nonself.[6] Unfortunately, this is a fairly common state. We can say, for example, that many of us have confused a relationship as something permanent, and when it spontaneously ends, we suffer. Or how often do we engage in activities that we find pleasurable—say, eating fast food, excessive partying, or having intensely dramatic romances—that years later we can look back on and with confidence say, *That really wasn't good for me,* even though at the time it felt good?

This state of confusion creates different layers of separation, within which lies the root of suffering. In the first example, the loss of the relationship we thought to be permanent, suffering is in the space between our expectation and our actual experience. The loss causes grief because what we thought was going to be no longer is, and we feel separate from our concept of what that relationship ought to have been; the world in our heads doesn't align with the external reality.

Much of the process of psychological maturation involves reflecting on instances when we engaged in activities that at the time we believed to be pleasurable, but, with the wisdom found in the passage of time, we now realize were actually detrimental. Although this is an oversimplification, many of us can relate to cycles of these types of behaviors in our lives. These create separation because they represent places and times when we were searching for ourselves, and taking refuge in the fleeting. As a result, we suffer. That suffering can be intense, even severe, as in the case of extreme loneliness or feelings of lostness that impair our ability to function properly. Or the suffering can be dull and manifest as a general dissatisfaction or sense of things not being quite right in our lives.

Observing the Laws

There are natural truths, laws by which this universe operates. In the physical, observable world we call them scientific or mathematical laws. On Earth, if you have an apple in your hand and you drop it, it will fall. It doesn't matter if you're in Japan or in Peru; gravitational pull will direct the apple toward Earth's core. There are laws everywhere: laws that are observation-based descriptions that tell us about the world we live in, laws that we can verify through experimentation and upon which we can make predictions about future states of being. There are laws in math and even laws that translate to art. If you mix blue and yellow together, you will get green. If you want to show three-dimensionality in a drawing, you must know how to work with perspective, how to draw objects in relation to one another and to their environment, like the way a set of train tracks drawn on paper seem to come together at the horizon.

When we come to understand these laws, we can learn to work with them so they become useful to us. We know how to make green on an artist's palette to paint tree leaves. Thanks to our understanding of physics, we can devise machines that will use gravity, instead of manpower, to move heavy objects. Similarly, there are laws of consciousness. The big one is this: The state of separation is the ultimate illusion.

Does saying that separation exists only in the imagination undermine my experiences of deep loneliness and confusion? Does it suggest that the pain I felt, the seemingly insurmountable sadness, was nothing more than mere delusion? No. It simply means those feelings were not *based* in reality or truth. Have you ever had a dream that someone you love did something terrible to you only to awaken and feel "legitimately" angry with them? The anger, that's real. But the person didn't actually do anything wrong; the anger is based on an illusion. That being said, illusions are powerful and can drive us to some interesting places, and separation seems to be a pervasive illusory state; everyone feels lonely, isolated, or depressed at some point or another. So if the state of separation is an illusion, what then is truth?

And Now, Yoga

Patañjali, the attributed author of the *Yoga Sūtras*, was a wordsmith. In 196 short statements, he managed to delineate the entire philosophy and practice of yoga. The man was concise. He makes Ernest Hemingway read like Charles Dickens. In an endeavor of such precision, every word matters. In the *Sūtras*, very much like in poetry, diction takes precedence: Every word is intentional. Additionally, every writer (and perhaps every reader) knows that the opening of a work must be strong to hook the reader, and the *Sūtras* are no exception. Furthermore, with so few words, each word must carry layers of meaning. Like poetry unfolding through metaphor, the *Sūtras* unravel layers of meaning with each statement.

Let's revisit the first *sūtra*: "Now, the teachings of yoga."[7]

Although the statement serves as an introduction on what's to come, there is no mistaking it: The first lesson lies right in front of us, in the very first word. The state of yoga is a revelation of what *really* matters—a lifting of a veil so that we may have accurate vision with which to see the world as it is. But where can we find yoga? The very first word of the *Sūtras* says it all: *Atha*—now. Yoga is always and exclusively available in the present moment. That is it.

Yoga is the actual state of reality. Yoga is the glasses coming off, that precious *aha!* moment of 20/20 vision—not in hindsight, but right here, where we stand.

As a word whose etymological meaning is to bind or yoke, we asked earlier of yoga, *What is being united?* Everything at once. Nothing at all. This is the paradox of our existence, and what keeps things interesting. Yoga isn't some sort of force that brings everything together; there is no means–ends relationship (if I do this, then this other great thing will happen; if I play nice and give money to the poor, then I'm going to heaven). That's not what's at stake. Yoga is the experience of everything coming into clarity in the moment at hand.

What does that mean, practically? We don't tend to live here, for the most part. We may think we're sitting in a New York City café in the present day, but in our heads, we're reliving the scene of that awful breakup back in California, eight years ago, or replaying that horrible argument from the night before. Often, we aren't fully aware of where we spend most of our mental time, and which thoughts we're "hanging out with" most. When we pay attention, we notice that the mental playgrounds we frequent tend to be cyclical. We repeat patterns, go back to certain memories or forward to certain fears or aspirations. Similarly, we may just be replaying the laundry list of our to-dos in our brains. But we don't often abide in the place where we take in the moment as it transpires.

In activities such as sports, music, dance, art, and running, the experience of yoga happens easily, because these require our presence; there is a level of concentration that draws us into the moment. Yoga is when the basketball leaves your hands and is headed straight for the net. It's landing that eight-point turn or the aerial dance step. It's the guitar, drum, or improvised trumpet jazz solo. It's realizing that three hours have gone by since you first picked up the pen, pencil, paintbrush, and you're still going. It's the instant you meet your beloved's eyes and everything else dissipates. It's feeling your child's breath deepen as he or she dozes off, nestled against your chest. These moments have something in common, and they're worth exploring. In these moments, we say we are in flow, we feel alive, we are in the zone, and they bring us pure joy. In these moments, we are open, free, and clear. Think back on how many of your most cherished memories are those when you were completely engaged in the moment. This is yoga: a happy accident and medicine for the heart.

As a healing form, the first *sūtra* also suggests that the answers to everything we seek are in front of us. This is the yogi's journey: an immersion in the present moment through an exploration of what is keeping us from being with what's here right now. This isn't easy; instead, it's a foray into our deepest experiences and our sense of identity. It's a project that requires gusto and guts. Yet, if we choose to walk the path of examination, filled with all its challenges, setbacks, obstacles, tears, frustrations, and countless times when we almost give up, we might find that not just our practical lives but our intrinsic sense of self can be radically transformed. This changes everything. If we choose to open that door and take the subsequent steps outside, what we find is an opportunity to touch the open expanse of true freedom—the basis for the deepest and sweetest of loves. The path of yoga is ultimately a journey home: to the present and to ourselves, unveiled.

5
THE WOUND
AND THE STORY

I can remember the first time I encountered the notion that I was not my anxiety, my sadness, or my thoughts. Though I had no idea what that meant, it came down on me like a sack of flour. I sat at my desk in my hallway-like room in Bushwick. The width of the room could barely hold a twin-sized bed and a small nightstand, but when I lay on my bed, the room seemed to stretch out to the horizon, ending in a miniature bathroom whose light I left on at night to protect me from the dark (a fear I'd had since childhood). On my desk, stacks of library books towered on either side of my computer and shadowed its screen. The little black cursor on the plain white computer background blinked furiously at me. I was immersed in research and writing for my graduate thesis on continental philosophy. I had been working on several chapters on the notion of *dasein*—a philosophy of being. I was getting nowhere.

I looked at the clock: 3:25 A.M. I couldn't write. I couldn't sleep. I was smothered in a blanket of anxiety that masked an underlying layer of pure, unadulterated sadness. The later (or earlier) it got, the less I could use work as a distraction from the growing pressure in my chest, the ticking time bomb I'd been carrying inside me. I got up to stretch and saw the book. I'd picked it up at a secondhand bookstore on my way home from class earlier that week and had started to read it on the train. *You are not your thoughts.* I'd underlined the sentence twice in red ink, though I couldn't quite grasp the meaning of this statement. In the academy, most of what I'd been taught was that my identity was exactly that: my thoughts—especially in the field of philosophy. Perhaps this is why that sentence captured me immediately.

I put the book down, tightened the blue bandana on my head—careful not to touch my hairline—and took another drag from my cigarette. I blew a few wobbly, empty rings into the air. The smoke lingered in the space around me and hovered around my lamp, adding to the surreal nature of the wee hours. I set the cigarette down and attempted another sentence of the document in front of me. Nothing came out. My fingers lay limp over the keyboard; my eyelids were heavy and tired. I looked at the keyboard once again and realized it was covered in hair.

I was rarely aware of when it happened anymore—the pulling—though I can pinpoint almost the exact moment it started. It was shortly after Mami's diagnosis. I was thirteen years old. Not long after her chemotherapy began, I'd catch the thinning strands of Mami's hair as they fell from her head. At first, it was only when I brushed her hair, but after a while, all it took was a gentle stroke and her once lush, healthy tresses would float into the air like dandelion spores.

Before the chemo, we called her *leona*, the lioness; that mane was her pride. I'd never seen hair like that, so thick it was fury and anarchy on her head. As a little girl, I'd fall asleep scratching Mami's head, dozing off with my tiny fingers lost in that midnight-black jungle. No one in the family had hair like Mami; not even my kinky curls came close. But her mane was no match for the chemo; it didn't even put up a fight. It just gave up the way the leaves surrender to the heaviness of winter, leaving trees bare without a choice. Toward the end, I'd catch full clumps of her hair at once. Patch by patch her soft skin revealed itself until there was nothing left to cover it. I remember her head smelling like a baby's. Mami was thirty-nine and on her last bare-headed, bare-tree winter when I started to unconsciously pull out my own hair.

My left hand fingered the keyboard while my right felt the contours of the bald spots covered by the bandana. Through high school and even college I'd learned more or less to control the tendency to pull. I devised techniques like sitting on my hands to braiding anything I could, like the strands at the end of a winter scarf or the paper covers over straws, anytime the tendency to pull called me. I even learned to shift the location of the pulling. If I caught myself fingering my hairline, I'd redirect my hands to my arms and legs, where the pulling would be substantially less fulfilling, but the remaining bald spots would be much less noticeable. Occasionally, my fingers would take a detour toward my eyebrows and eyelashes, as though fighting me for a compromise. I figured I could always put on mascara and brush in my eyebrows, so I let my restriction slide from time to time.

Come my freshman year of college, I tried a more dire strategy and cut off nearly twenty inches of my ringlets, leaving very little hair on my head I could play with. The rest I covered with a red bandana that I tied tightly to my scalp, blockading my sneaky little digits, which appeared to have developed a mind of their own. Like a tropical storm that's made its passage through land and, once satisfied, returns to the sea, the irresistible hunger to pull out my own hair began to fade until it seemed to disappear. Seemed to. I thought: *Well, thank God that's over.* In truth, the beast was hibernating. Dormancy is not equivalent to healing, but I didn't know that then.

During my first winter in New York City, the bizarre tic reawakened as though carried in by the overwhelming tide of the season's sadness, as though it were foreshadowing the descent that was still to come. Like seaweed, the sadness began to wrap itself around my ankles and started to pull me under, but I didn't notice what was happening. I was unaware I was drowning. I only noticed the displaced strands of individual curls around the computer keyboard, the mouse, my lap, and the balding spots expanding across my cranium, my eyelashes and eyebrows receding, revealing baby-soft skin.

Trichotillomania is a rare form of obsessive-compulsive disorder characterized by the urge to pull out one's own hair. Its onset is between the ages of nine and thirteen, and it is often set off by trauma. The condition can appear and then disappear. It can lie dormant until it's re-triggered, often by stressful events. I learned this after the fact—after the hair on my head, eyelashes, and eyebrows started growing back. In retrospect, it makes perfect sense that an unconscious and uncontrollable urge to pull out my own hair would arise as I watched my mother's thick tresses fall away.

It would also make sense that I would develop anorexia during this same period, as I watched my mother's once voluptuous body dwindle to bones. At thirteen, I did not have the ability or tools to consciously comprehend or integrate what was happening to Mami, and my psyche and body compensated by reacting in ways that were somehow parallel to what Mami was going through. A tangled form of empathy evolved; I managed my own experience by developing coping mechanisms that would require over a decade to understand and longer to truly heal. In the middle of my newfound loneliness in New York, the trichotillomania and disordered eating were re-triggered. These weren't the only things that decided to wake up and be seen in broad daylight.

The OCD was just one layer, one veil or story. The sadness was another. The loneliness one more. Much like Russian nesting dolls, we tend to live encased in covers, one inside the other, covers we create like papier-mâché, so they harden and are able to protect the most vulnerable and gentle, the softest and most precious of all the things we have: our hearts.

The Protecting Sheath

In the practice of *haṭha yoga* we know that if a part of the body is injured, other parts of the body will react around it, compensating for and shielding it like a defensive force. Consequently, inflammation might occur in the surrounding muscles and ligaments to guard against further injury. The body, physically as well as emotionally and spiritually, protects itself by creating sheaths so that the hurt part of us—be it a hamstring or a childhood experience—can heal. In so doing, the injury can be said to contract and construct a shell around itself.

In the physical body, we see this principle at play in the example of a cut. When you nick a finger chopping vegetables, the cut will throb as the blood rushes to the spot it needs to protect. You place gauze over the cut, and apply pressure. It feels as though your heart is right at the center of the cut, and your attention is drawn to that space. It seems larger, and suddenly that new body part gains a different type of awareness. Whereas in your day-to-day life you wouldn't normally think too much about the inner surface of your left middle finger, after the cut you pay attention to shield it. What you do and the way you think and move change because of it. You might decide not to play basketball the next day, as you'd originally planned. Or if you do play, you avoid dribbling with that hand, as a hyperawareness of the wounded space develops. This may seem obvious, but remember that the philosophical and ontological task at hand is to examine what we take for granted and do habitually, for therein lie interesting lessons. The lesson here is that our attention is naturally drawn to our wounds, and that our choices, relationships, and even the way we move through the world can start revolving around them.

Emotionally, we function similarly. When we are in emotional pain, we contract—that is to say, we tighten and create layers that protect us from the outside world. In the tightening, all the surrounding areas (e.g., our relationships, our long-term goals, etc.) become secondary and the pain primary. The pain becomes what we see; we experience everything else *through* it. For a while, it may be all we can think about, and our reality becomes the layers we have created for our protection.

Take, for example, someone who has experienced unfaithfulness in a romantic partnership. Say also that the person who committed the betrayal recognizes their mistake, sincerely apologizes, and promises never to do it again. Even if both parties have the best of intentions to move forward, in the period following the affair, the betrayed partner will be especially sensitive and will be easily reminded of the lost trust. A phone call past a certain time, the mention of a particular name, or an innocent comment can feel more consequential than it is and is a reminder of their wounded heart. The hurt partner may become hypervigilant and unable to relax. The nervous system is turned on and all senses are awakened, hyperalert to potential danger. During this time, while the wound is fresh, the hurt partner is experiencing life contracted, and life *through* the experience of the wound itself. The betrayal is the primary lens through which the hurt party is interpreting reality at that time.

If we are mindful and healthy, then time, friends, community, hobbies, and life moving on will help us to expand once again. Occasionally, it's a long, long time, and much of it depends on what we already have to work with internally; namely, how much work we've already done in relation to our past wounding. As we relearn to open, we can see the world through a different lens, and the pain occupies less space in our experience. In the example of the relationship betrayal, the hurt partner may look at their partner and start seeing their desirable traits again, instead of the unfaithfulness. Rebuilding can begin, even with the potential of creating stronger bonds than the ones originally present, because a tough battle has been overcome together. In the example of cutting our finger while cooking, the Band-Aid eventually comes off and we go back to playing basketball the way we once did. The wound gets some air, and although it is perhaps a little sore, we stop protecting it, and our attention is drawn in the direction of other interests.

Sometimes, however, it's not so easy: We leave the Band-Aid on the wound for far longer than it needs to be there. We overprotect, refuse to give it fresh air, or even choose to ignore it without first tending to it; a new layer of skin grows, much like the roots of a tree may grow around the bricks and asphalt that surround them. When we don't heal the wound and instead layer our lives over it, the wound becomes part of us. This sore, emotional scar is embedded in the story of how we believe the world functions, and who we imagine ourselves to be. The wound doesn't go away; it remains hidden and blocked, and it grows numb behind all that protection. We may become unaware of it, or forget it ever existed at all.

The Fabricating Veil

We all wear many hats. These hats depend on whom we are with, what tasks we are in the middle of accomplishing, and how we want to show up in the world. Each hat comes with its own story. Every story we tell is made up of experiences, ambitions, places, and people who have crossed our path and are meaningful to us. Every story creates a layer of our ego, our ego being our means of self-identification, what we believe separates us and makes us unique from everything else around us. The ego is our own sense of self.

Problems occur when many of these stories, and especially our wound stories, go unchecked and we identify ourselves with them; when we forget that we are writers of a story and dictators of our own narrative. The problem also arises when we write and rewrite the stories of who we are and how we came to be without awareness that we are doing so. Often, we compose these stories not out of the best material, of the parts of ourselves that are most aware and alive, but out of what we fear most or are trying to hide from the world, and perhaps from ourselves.

It's common knowledge that eyewitness testimonials are one of the least reliable sources of evidence. Twenty people can see the same scene and offer twenty different versions of what they think happened, all based on that person's angle, outlook, and means of understanding the world. Stories are powerful tools, so much so that every civilization has had its own set to explain the inexplicable, whether that be the creation of the world or why it rains in the springtime. Every culture has its myths and fables, and many of the great prophets spoke in stories, parables, and allegories. We are, by nature, story-telling people, and it is the stories we tell ourselves *about ourselves* that are the most powerful, and potentially the most perilous of all—especially when we are naïve to our own flavor of storytelling. Our stories describe the way we see the world, and in so doing, we create our world around our stories.

When we are in the story, we are not in our hearts. Instead, we are in our heads, living in the fabricated veil that keeps us both from healing and from living a life authentic to who we truly are and what is actually in front of us. The ego stories, when unbridled, most often serve to create a sense of separation within us, a trance of identity that keeps us in a space of suffering. Some scholars, such as Edwin Bryant, suggest that the dull form of suffering—that pervasive feeling of dissatisfaction with life, work, friends, or partners—is more like a frustration, one that comes at our attempt to find satisfaction in that which is temporary. Again, we're confusing the temporary or unreal with the permanent or real. But there's also the acute suffering that might appear as depression, anxiety, or other ailments that make life a true struggle.

Yet, who are we really, if not our stories? In philosophical and psychological debates regarding personal identity, it has been proposed that one of the elements that distinguishes human consciousness from that of animals or artificial intelligence may be our ability to create autobiographies. There *is* something unique about the way our human mind works in relationship to how we perceive ourselves in time and in relation to everything and everyone else in our sphere of consciousness. Namely, we take events from our lives and link them together in such a way as to create a linear narrative with a clear star of the show, as well as main and supporting characters. In this way, we construct a set of connections and meaning that to some degree we feel defines us—or more accurately, that we define ourselves by.

This is where yoga comes in. Again, yoga happens when all the hats come off. Underneath everything we've done, every person we've met, and every story we've told ourselves is a primordial identity, unmasked. Underneath the sheaths of action, desire, pain, and striving is simply being-ness. Yoga is the realization—the awareness of and connectedness to the simplicity of unmasked being—and the collection of practices that helps us to, perhaps momentarily, remember what we already know: that all else aside, we simply *are*. The message is straightforward and almost simplistic; but it's also powerful. It turns out that, whereas we are exceptionally good at doing and at associating with our doing-ness (i.e., identifying ourselves by our careers, or what we produce, or what we've accomplished), we're not so great at just being—without titles, identities, or labels.

Yet, it's this simple being-ness that we share with everything else that exists, from our siblings to our companion animals and even a water bottle. Everything, in its simplest form, simply is, regardless of its degree of sentience. The qualitative nature of aliveness, the different sensations of being, and the degree of consciousness and self-consciousness shift from creature to creature. But being-ness in itself is the most universal, quintessential, and undeniable thing there is.

Yogic thought suggests that this awareness is part of our homecoming—remembering and connecting to the simplicity of aliveness—and it's precisely here that we find the ultimate expression of creativity, abundance, freedom, and love. Within the sphere of just being, the need for stories melts away. And so, through this remembrance of and connection to simple awareness, our stories twinkle like Christmas lights and we start seeing what was once dormant and habitual. Through practicing and tuning in to the simplicity of being, we bring awareness to the stories we compose. We start shedding our wounds and find healing and freedom.

Organizing and Cleaning Our "Stuff"

The application of yogic principles heals through work, not magic, and the *Yoga Sūtras* clearly lays out that work for us. It begins by creating awareness of the "stuff," the layers we have (unintentionally) created, perhaps as an attempt to protect unhealed wounds. My fight with trichotillomania OCD is one example of a wound left unchecked. As it had never been explored, it reawoke from dormancy because it wasn't fully healed (and hence I was not free from it).

Our task, then, on the yogic path is to delve into our layers and examine the sheaths that may have acted to shield us from the cold and pain but were never removed. When overlooked, the sheaths become like old luggage we schlep with us everywhere, even though we're running out of room. The bags are heavy as hell, and we're tired of carrying them. Yet, we unknowingly become hoarders of our stories and bring their heaviness to different relationships—whether with our friends, lovers, or ourselves—adding further to our baggage. All the while, we may be completely unaware of any of this.

Imagine if we cleaned the clutter! What might it be like if we neatly organized our boxes of music, properly displayed our stacks of photos in albums, folded our clothes and organized them in the closet according to style and season. Imagine if every cupboard and dresser in our homes were immaculate, the basement and attic spotless, and everything had its place. Imagine if we knew exactly where we kept each valuable memory, anecdote, and keepsake, and if all of them were dusted and unsoiled. Imagine if we were clean from the inside out.

The work of yoga is the same as the healing of yoga: organizing and cleaning out our stuff so we can see it all clearly. In doing so, we see ourselves clearly. The path of yoga asks us to come home to ourselves and meet what is there, in all its disheveled glory—a task much easier said than done. Thankfully, there are guidelines. The *Yoga Sūtras of Patañjali* is a map of the layers of the self, and a tool to help us navigate, organize, and get rid of the clutter we don't need so we can see what lies beneath. When we touch center, we arrive at our truest nature.[8]

6

THE TURNINGS
OF THE MIND

Commentators on the original Sanskrit text generally agree that the second *sūtra* is one of the most (if not the most) pivotal *sūtras* in the entire collection. It reads: "The restraint of the modifications of the mind-stuff is yoga."[9] Why is this *sūtra* so important? Because it explains the state of yoga as well as the conditions out of which it arises. It is the first and most important thing we need to know, and if there is only one thing for us to know, it is this: Yoga happens when the habitual gears stop turning. Yoga occurs in the absence of movement, in the creation of focus, and in the presence of presence.

For the most part, we live in a world of commotion and noise. Although a good portion of that world is external noise—the bustle of traffic, routine conversations, or the constant barrage of advertisements—the *Yoga Sūtras* is most interested in the internal noise, the movement in our minds. The two are, of course, related. External stimuli will create an internal response, much of it involuntary. The scent of a freshly baked brownie will immediately trigger recognition of the aroma and a pairing with a taste. Perhaps, too, it will arouse desire for the brownie, and maybe even stir up memories of your grandmother baking brownies and the love you felt for her as child. It might make you miss her and reach out for that brownie. Like Marcel Proust and his tasty madeleine, we savor the delectables with our senses, and they return us to fond moments and re-create them in the present. If, on the contrary, your first memory of a brownie is about having a terrible allergic reaction that sent you to the hospital, the result might be different. You might stay away from brownies in general.

Through the basic example of a brownie, we can gain some insight into the workings of the mind from the yogic perspective. And while the principles are simple, the implications are profound and can ultimately aid us in our path to healing and lasting happiness. The function of the mind from the yogic view follows a clear set of patterns. First, through what is referred to as *manas*, we take in stimuli through the sensory perception. Anything we are exposed to comes in through our eyes, ears, noses, touch receptors, or taste buds.

Secondly, the *buddhi*—the intellectual faculty responsible for discernment, intelligence, and reasoning—kicks in, meaning we decipher what things are based on our prior experience with that object. This is what allows us to distinguish between objects. Doing so arouses a storehouse of identifications with the objects we encounter (usually pleasant or unpleasant), which will determine the last part of the process: whether we want that brownie or not. Here, we have encountered the *ahaṅkāra*, ego, or our feeling of "I"-ness or individuation that creates in us the sense that we are distinct from everyone and everything else around us. When we reach desire, we do so because we have struck ego.

The sentence "I want _____" contains two necessary and interdependent aspects. You cannot have desire without ego, the notion of a discernible "I"; and you cannot have desire without the blank—the sense of lack that suggests the object of desire will fulfill that lack. When we look closely, yogic wisdom is not making a subtle point about the nature of desire here. On the contrary, desire (as well as its counterpart, aversion) from the yogic perspective is intertwined with our faculties of perception, meaning that we are likely to generate an aversion- or desire-type reaction to the environmental stimulus we are exposed to. On the other side of the coin, it is improbable (and perhaps impossible) that I will develop a desire or aversion to something I've never been exposed to.

So why does this matter? I'll use an example: I have never uttered the sentence, "I'm really craving frogs' legs right now," simply because I've never experienced eating frogs' legs. However, I've definitely said, "I could use some ice cream right now." Even after having given up all dairy products in my teens, memories of a smooth and cooling serving of vanilla ice cream on a summer day are still present with me, and on occasion I will crave ice cream. My ability to keep myself from eating dairy-based ice cream is now, decades after I first gave it up, far greater than it was a week after I decided to stop consuming dairy. Although I still retain memories of and positive associations with dairy ice cream, I am far removed from the action and habit of eating it by many years. The more distance between me and an action, the softer my craving will be and the easier it will be for me not to give in and partake in the object of desire. In other words, the fresher and stronger the impression of the ice cream is in my consciousness, the more likely it is I will be a victim of that impression. Likewise, the closer I am in time to the action I'm trying to avoid, the more difficult or rather the more *uncomfortable* the avoidance of that action will be. Desire, then, is a direct result of the stimuli that we are exposed to, or more accurately, the stimuli we choose to expose ourselves to.

I'd like to draw attention to the experience of desire for a moment—the bodily discomfort of craving, the sensation for longing, and the perception of lack associated with wishing to fulfill a desire. Experientially speaking, a desire for ice cream, soda, a different job, or a romantic relationship are all rooted in our experiences of the world, and all have a particular sensation in our physical bodies. The more we indulge in the object of the desire, and the more complex our stories around that desire are, the deeper the habit or the impression perpetuated in our minds. This impression then circles back to our (often unconscious) choices.

The cycle of desire/aversion is a driving force for the ceaseless mind-chatter that keeps us from being present and at ease—fully in yoga, in presence. Desire/aversion is one of the strongest drivers not only of our behavior but our sense of identity, and consequently the situations we create and re-create for ourselves. In essence, desire/aversion becomes a push/pull that can drastically affect the quality of our lives.

And here we have come full circle. From the scent of a brownie we arrive at one of the most essential quandaries of the human condition: the problem of lack or suffering. Most of the problem happens in the backdrop of thought, unnoticed. Yet, we can become aware of it when we are in the throes of suffering from an unfulfilled desire—the irresistible pull to the brownie, the cigarette, the piece of cake, or the ex whose number we still have on speed dial. Otherwise, we feel it's due to aversion when we are strongly repelled by a situation, when we feel like we just have to run away. This is our deep conditioning; whether it's desire or aversion, we repeat the cycle: We fall off the wagon, get back on the wagon, make promises to ourselves, break those promises, and repeat on loop until we finally become dizzy enough to say: *This has got to stop.*

Round and Round We Go: The Story and Its Perpetuation

Yoga is interested in drawing attention to the cyclical nature of the "turnings of the mind," to transform those very turnings. When we pay attention, we notice that our daily thought patterns are habitual and repetitive in nature. We tend to think/obsess/daydream about the same things over and over. Whether it's in list-making form, an ongoing monologue, or repetitive images in the mind, these thought patterns create a trancelike state that affects how we experience life and how we show up in the world. The more the same thoughts are thought, the more likely we are to continue thinking them. In other words, our thought patterns become deeply entrenched habits that are increasingly difficult to change the longer we keep them. Indeed, thought patterns can be so habitual that they sit outside our spectrum of awareness. We are like the fish who's the last to find out what water is.

We can't expect behavior to stray too far from our state of mind, for how we act reflects (though oftentimes is more like a reaction to) our state of mind and the thoughts that we choose to give time and space to within our consciousness. Hence, the result of cyclical thinking is cyclical action: We do the same things over and over; we make the same mistakes and become consumed in our habits. This may manifest differently in different areas of our lives. Perhaps it's the diet plan we have attempted time and again with little to no success; or maybe it's that despite the different jobs we have had, we always find ourselves getting taken advantage of by our superiors; or many of us have dated the "same" person in several different bodies, only to end up thinking *Here I am again*, and feeling as though our circumstances will never change. We feel like our lives are out of our control, as though life itself keeps presenting the same obstacles repeatedly in some twisted game: *I've been through this already. Why does this keep happening to me?*

Feelings of victimhood further contribute to the issue, and these experiences amount in effect to the creation of a story about who we are: *I am the person who can never give up pizza; I am the person who always dates the bad boys/the unfaithful women; I will always be a hot mess.* The story is an attempt to tie our varied experiences into a neat little package that can account for why things are the way they are in our lives. The story also effectively takes responsibility out of our hands. For if something is the way it is intrinsically, there's not much to be done about it. So, we continue like a mouse on its wheel. As the story gets told and retold, both to others and ourselves, it weaves itself further into the fabric of who we believe ourselves to be. In this way, we create ourselves and our limitations.

Spiritual growth is about taking responsibility for the person we have made ourselves to be, and the person we continue creating in each moment, with each choice, physical or non-physical. It requires a delicate balance of (in the words of the sages) restraint—the restraint that is integral to the very definition of yoga, which must also be met, as we will soon learn, with a healthy dose of surrender.

Underlying both these elements is the first step of our growth: witnessing. Only through witnessing can we take inventory of what's there, and become aware of what we have to work with. The more we witness, the more we learn. The second step is restraint. By restraint, the sages are not necessarily referring to an ascetic sensibility. Instead, restraint is about a cultivation of discipline with the mind, and with the stories we tell ourselves that develop fundamental belief systems that we unconsciously abide by and that end up directing our behavior. When a fundamental belief about the way life works continues to repeat itself in our thoughts, the world appears through that lens. The problem with this circular patterning is that we then come to mistakenly believe that life works within the parameters we have constructed, and as such, life seems to controls us; we feel dominated by life's mysterious forces, subjected to the same patterns that present themselves repeatedly. Stepping into spiritual maturation requires that we learn to discern that which we can control, and that which we cannot. It is the former that requires restraint, and the latter that necessitates surrender.

7
A PLACE TO CALL HOME

We lived out of our car. I was ten years old. It was almost two years after Papi's passing back in Colombia, but he and Mami were from different social classes and after his death his whole family shunned my mother. Whereas Mami had barely graduated high school and most of her family had only completed grade school, Papi's family was made up of engineers, professors, and lawyers. Papi, too, was an engineer, and a talented musician. He'd left behind a house, an engineering firm, a library of books that ranged from Carl Sagan's work to the autobiography of the fourteenth Dalai Lama, and a collection of classical instruments.

Papi was killed in a head-on collision with a drunk driver, two days before his thirty-seventh birthday. Papi's family, who considered my mother too uneducated and therefore unfit to carry my father's lineage, saw to it that none of his life's work remained with Mami. With the help of expensive lawyers and a crooked legal system that Mami had no means to fight against, we lost everything within a year. The family fought to take my younger sister, Vannesa, and me from her as well, but she won that battle. Mami had family in the States, so we found ourselves with only two suitcases' worth of belongings, an old used car, and Papi's Brazilian classical guitar left to our names as we tried to find a home in the San Francisco Bay Area. We lived out of our car and slept in sleeping bags or on a relative's couch until an uncle cleared out part of his garage and allowed us to stay there.

The rats were huge, easily the size of small cats. This is what I remember most about the garage. They made loud squealing noises, curled up in the crevices behind the kitchen sink, and scurried in our dresser drawers during the night. Two-thirds of the garage floor was covered by carpet samples, each a different color, pattern, and texture. The rest of the floor was exposed, cold and hard. There were no windows. We had to be cautious not to touch the uncovered pink insulation or the red, blue, and black wires that lined the inside walls. Its single toilet worked sparingly. We had to let the water run brown for several minutes before the tap in the kitchen sink released clear liquid. And if more than two appliances were plugged in simultaneously, the electricity would short and the lights would inevitably go out.

Behind the garage was a rickety wire fence with slender pieces of rotten wood that ran through it like decaying bars on a holding cell. The splintery panels failed to conceal the silhouette of a hefty metal refinery behind those bars, separated only by an expanse of gravel. This is where the rats came from. Giant pipes extended into the sky like massive steel arms and released a dark and musky smoke into the sky.

Mami, only thirty-three when my father passed, worked several jobs. She cleaned houses, had a janitorial position at an antique-porcelain store, attended night school to learn English at the local junior college, and volunteered as an art teacher at our little public school in West San Jose. One Sunday morning, Mami bought a can crusher at a garage sale down the street from us, and from that day forward, Mami, Vannesa, and I developed a new ritual. On Sunday evenings, after weekends had been celebrated and dinners eaten, but before the weekly morning garbage collection, the three of us drove through the wealthier regions of the South Bay: Saratoga, Willow Glen, Palo Alto. We passed row upon row of lavishly colonnaded, multi-bedroomed houses, with expansive porches strung with colorful hammocks, and backyards lined with trees. On the street in front of the homes were mountains of black bags filled with their garbage, unsupervised.

Lucky for us, one thing the inhabitants of these palaces had in common was that they enjoyed their soda. In cans. Mami, Vannesa, and I would each take an empty bag and rummage for cans of Coca-Cola and Pepsi, Sprite and Dr Pepper, sometimes Budweiser. We'd turn it into a game, counting the reds and silvers, blues and greens; who could collect more of which, who could beat out whom. We'd bring the bags home and crush them in the small machine, then refill our bags. The next day after school, we'd take our aluminum treasures to the recycling station, where, after weighing each bag, we'd get cash, just like that. Ten, fifteen, sometimes even twenty dollars. We'd drive home, smiling brightly. Once home, Mami would often say to me in her pensive manner, "Life is hard, *hija*; but it's worth it."

Mami eventually saved enough money for us to leave the garage and move into a small apartment in West San Jose, off Pedro Street, behind the freeway. Compared to the garage, it was a Victorian castle. The bedroom and the living room both had windows! A single carpet covered the whole apartment, no patches. The electricity and water worked, the bathroom toilet flushed, more than two appliances could be plugged in at any given time, and we even had working heat! As we began moving our few belongings in, we realized: *This could be home, this could* really *be home.*

Before long, we found our Pedro Street community: Araceli next door, and Jerry with his impeccably pressed khakis, wife-beater, and red bandana hanging from his pocket down in Apartment 1; the Martinez brother and sister, the same ages as Vannesa and me, at the end of the block. On summer days, we'd splash each other with running water from the green garden hose, and play hide-and-seek in and out of garages, ringing on doorbells and running off in a frenzy. The hot sun tanned our faces and our clear jelly flip-flops blistered our feet, but we were too excited to feel them hurt. The longer the sun stayed with us, the longer we could enjoy *la calle*, our street, our own Pedro Street, before heading in and locking the door behind us at the first sign of the moon.

As soon as the sun went down, Pedro Street and its surrounding areas revealed their dark side. After nightfall, West San Jose was no place to walk alone. At the sight of the moon, *los pandilleros* arose like famished vampires. Their desire for blood wasn't metaphorical. Different streets in the same three-mile radius were claimed by different gangs: the *Sureños*, the *Norteños*, and the Bloods. On certain nights, the wind grew cold and whispers spread that the *Sureños* were taking heads, or the Bloods were in search of virgins. Sirens were a natural part of the soundtrack of the neighborhood, and popping gunshots became easy to ignore after the first year.

El Dorado, our local public school, turned out to be a breeding ground for the illegitimate children of gang members. They were kids who dressed in clothes five times their size, Dickies carefully starched, belts with letters and numbers on them that signified belonging, and shirts either red, blue, or black. El Dorado had its own uniform; it also had its own mother tongue. The children of this land spoke in riddled hand motions, a sign language of crooked fingers and disturbing symbols whose mere appearance felt threatening. Signs were not made; they were thrown like staccato punches, as if firing invisible weapons, squeezing multiple silent triggers.

The school was small and poor, consisting of a single administrative building with three trailers out back, and a lone basketball pole on the blacktop. Teachers came and went each year, sometimes each quarter. Familiar adult faces were few, and many looked young and intimidated; the white ones, particularly the females, never lasted long. Vannesa's graduating class (if you can call it that, since most children didn't graduate but moved on to continuation schools, juvenile halls, or back out to the streets) was notorious for the number of teachers that came and went. They were young souls who thought they could take on seventh graders from a bad part of town and teach them, help them grow, and show them a better, brighter way of life. They found themselves drowning in an ocean of handmade tattoos, marijuana smoke, brass-knuckled knives worn like trophies, vodka-spiked orange juice, and threats about fathers and uncles in jail who could and would make the teacher disappear if they didn't comply with the student's demands. In seventh grade alone, Vannesa's class went through eight teachers, each one leaving afraid, and almost never with two weeks' notice. Substitutes were more the rule than the exception.

My eighth-grade class had thirteen girls, including myself. Only three of us were virgins and only four of us didn't have tattoos across our budding young breasts. These displayed bold roman numerals—**XIII, XIV**—or the names of lovers or family lost to violence or jail time splayed across necks and backs, and surrounded by deliberate black and blues: some bruises, some hickeys. All loudly claimed ownership. However, we all wore the mandatory dark-brown lipliner around our little mouths like serious, angry clowns.

I honestly can't remember how many gang-initiation fights I witnessed on that blacktop behind the seventh-grade trailers. Most of them went something like this: Boys would shake hands with fists and pointed fingers. Then, with only a nod from the leader, the group surrounded the initiate—a boy of thirteen, fourteen at most—and descended on him like vultures encircling prey. Once the first punch was laid, a barrage followed. Soon, the boy's brow was bleeding profusely as he curled into a fetal position to protect his vital organs. Once down, the kicks ensued, steel-toed shoes slamming into the boy's legs, head, back, and ribs. He'd moan inadvertently, one arm covering his face, the other hugging his knees tightly—just a boy, a boy trying to be a man, while the gang's leader counted (*sixteeeen . . . fifteeeen . . .*) the seconds the child would have to survive to be accepted. Each second seemed to expand into hours. *When is it ending?* I thought every single time. The girls watched, fingers clutching the chain-link fence, half of us—the newbies—appalled, holding one another's hands or covering our mouths. The other half were unfazed, even rooting for the boy or those assaulting him. I can see them today: the young girls with their hands on one hip, a loosie dangling from the side of their lips, mouths framed by lipliner, joining their smoke and profanities with the kid's groans and grunts.

When it ended, when the leader's count finally hit zero, everything stopped, as if in a movie. And then it was quiet and still. The boy was on the ground, his body moving only so he could breathe. "You're done," the leader would say, and the boy on the blacktop shifted, revealing a swollen face, bits of gravel in his wounds, his lips and teeth concealed by blood, and his once-white T-shirt stained.

"Welcome to the family, homie."

One December, about a week before Christmas, Mami took Vannesa and me out of school to help her at work. She had three houses to clean that day. By the time we reached the third house, Mami looked more exhausted than usual. She was especially quiet. While I dusted Mr. Trainor's study, a sock rag and Pledge in hand, I heard a strange sound coming from the adjacent room. When I went to investigate, I realized it was Mami vomiting in the bathroom. That Christmas Eve, Mami lost consciousness and was rushed to the hospital, where she underwent extensive testing followed by an emergency operation. The operation revealed late-stage pancreatic cancer, which had metastasized rapidly throughout her body. She was given three weeks to live. Mami was put on a hearty regimen of radiation and chemotherapy, and her body seemed to diminish exponentially with each passing day.

Tending for Mami during her illness was like watching a time-lapse video, only each moment is both expanded and yet over too soon. Each day was filled with both gratitude for the borrowed time and fear it could be the last time we said goodnight, or the last time we kissed her soft face or looked into her huge, dark eyes. In these moments, every instant became precious and unique, as though funneled through a prism that revealed the simple divinity of each minute spent by her side. A single laugh from Mami indicated a second of relief from her ceaseless pain, and that was enough of a reason to celebrate. The little things meant everything.

Vannesa and I missed most of the remainder of that school year and stayed home to take care of Mami with the help of a relative, as we didn't have the means to hire medical staff. Mami could no longer perform the most basic tasks on her own. We fed her, since she could no longer eat solid foods; her only intake was through a tube that was placed in her stomach after surgery. We walked her, since she lost her ability to move without assistance almost immediately and was consistently hooked up to the feeding machine and a morphine IV drip, which Vannesa and I also administered carefully. We changed her, washed her clothes, gave her sponge baths, and massaged her emaciated body.

Overnight, my little sister and I, at twelve and thirteen, became our mother's primary caretakers and our world became a measured and recorded one: of numbers, charts, and fluid ounces. Every hour was calibrated and computed, spent notating every single one of Mami's changes, intakes, and bodily emissions. It was like taking care of a delicate and intricate machine. We measured eight ounces of Ensure through the stomach tube every four hours; logged temperature changes and ejections (vomit, urine); and recorded her moods, hours slept, and amount of morphine in her IV drip. This is how we tried to buy time: through precise calculation. We racked up any extra minutes at her side, and loved her as much as we could in these borrowed moments. At night, Vannesa and I would watch Mami sleep, her face peaceful after the morphine kicked in. We'd sit by her side, each one holding either of her hands, and say prayers together. We'd offer all the things we owned—our little apartment, our few toys, our own lives—to God, the Virgin Mary, and any saints who happened to be listening, if they would please not take her from us. Part of us believed in that magic; that life might just work like that, in precious wagers.

Mami lived four months past her diagnosis. She died in our arms on a beautiful afternoon in late May, a few days after Mother's Day. I remember looking out the window of her hospital room. I remember the sound of birds chirping and observing the way the flower blossoms seemed to float into the clouds, as if all of them knew there was a leaving. I remember her body seemed lighter when she passed. I remember when her body began to change hue. I remember the moment I knew she was no longer there.

I was fourteen years old.

8

THE TRUTH BEHIND OUR STORIES

Life's Ruthless Colors

I can say that these stories used to possess me, as I can honestly admit that there still lies some remnants of attachment, of *This is who I am; this is what I've been through,* within me in relation to the CliffsNotes of how I immigrated to the United States, lived in substandard and unsafe conditions, took care of my mother on her last days, and became an orphan before even entering high school. Yet, in truth I didn't become fully aware that I carried the heaviness of my story with me everywhere—in both heart and body—until I began to delve into yogic work. I didn't realize that these stories had become my identity and drenched me in a sorrow that owned me for many years. Nor did I realize these narratives were how *I understood myself.* I didn't have the clarity to see the patterns that I'd re-create years later, like in my twenties when the only men I was attracted to were those with gang-affiliated tattoos covering their necks, the words **THUG LIFE** in Old English across their abdomen. It was when the yogic work truly began that I started to glimpse another truth altogether.

In reality, my story is like any other story: a metaphor. A metaphor simultaneously highlights and hides. Every time we choose to tell a story (whether to others or ourselves), we are (deliberately or subconsciously) choosing a particular focus. But there are always myriad foci. Some theorists also believe that metaphors are a more accurate representation of our human experience than referential language. Our experience is multifaceted and language is limited. When we speak referentially, we can say a word like *tree* and every person in the room who has seen a tree will have a clear object in their mind. Yet, two issues arise. First, what are the chances that every person is think-ing of the same type of tree? Slim to none; each person's image of a tree is dependent on their experiences of trees. Conducting this very exercise in my philosophy classes, I get, without fail, a vast assortment of trees—ranging from pines to weeping wil-lows—all demonstrative of the experiences of the people in the class.

The second issue is this: If the notion of a tree—a very basic object in the world—can elicit such a wide assortment of visual and emotional memories, what then of more abstract concepts, like happiness, faith, truth, or love? This thought experiment sheds light on a fundamental epistemological question: How much can we really communicate if our experiences are all so different?

The truth about reality that yoga philosophy opens us to is that there are endless outlooks and potentially infinite ways to apprehend a situation or story. In my case, with the limited understanding of a child, what I took my story to mean—how I interpreted my own experience—was epitomized in my mother's own words: *Life is hard.* I saw that axiom reflected in the radical shift of our lifestyle, from comfort to poverty in under a year; in my mother's grief after losing a partner she'd been with for nearly two decades; in her struggle to make ends meet, and despite her best efforts, never succeeding in the traditional way, never fulfilling that American Dream; and then in her sudden illness and death at such a young age. From that point of view, my mother's story—of an immigrant widow who had to leave her children to fend for themselves in an unforgiving world—is truly tragic. When I looked back and as I looked forward, all I could see was suffering and struggle: How would I make it in the world without parents? How would I support myself and care for my sister? How would we ever get out of poverty? Struggle. Life was going to be hard. I knew it. And I was right. My life only got harder.

Life's ruthless colors continued to reveal themselves to me after my mother's pass-ing and my experiences in the throes of legal guardianship. My teenage years were volatile to say the least: riddled with messy court hearings, moving from one foster home to another, fighting deportation, entering and exiting schools, and ultimately living in a home where it simply wasn't safe for a child.

A few weeks after Mami's passing, Vannesa and I left West San Jose and moved in with our guardians to a little town nestled in the Sierra foothills, about three hours north of the city. Once again, our circumstance had dictated that we must leave home. This time, without Mami.

Our primary guardians were unstable; they used force, threats, intimidation, and coercion to establish discipline. Although my sister and I may have had a roof over our heads, we were once again without a home in a foundational sense. We were emotionally displaced.

It didn't take long for our guardians to reveal their guardianship style when they decided we were not allowed to keep in touch with our friends from back home. Any letters we received would be confiscated, and any we tried to mail out would also be taken from us. Once school started, we were not allowed to see new friends after school or over the weekends; we were to have very little connection to the outside world.

Once, my guardian found a note in my backpack that my friend Rachelle had written to me on the school bus. The note used the word *shit*. My guardian made me sit in a chair while she berated me, telling me I was no good and that I'd never amount to anything, and that my sister and I deserved all the punishment life had given us: it was our fault our parents died. Our punishments never seemed to fit our crimes.

Within weeks, anxiety and terror began to take over. My guardians' footsteps down the long hallway that led to our room were enough to make my skin crawl. I feared waking up in the morning to find I had done something "wrong," often to be tossed into a bathroom and have the door shut on me. My guardians were obsessed with cleaning and frequently forced my sister and me to clean kitchen and bathroom floors with toothbrushes until two in the morning, or they would wake us up from our sleep in the middle of the night if something had not been done to their liking.

On too many days, I hid my sore and peeling hands in my pockets at school for fear that someone would notice their redness, the way the cleaning chemicals had burned my skin because they'd been submerged for too long. If the dusting wasn't done right, if a knickknack was more than a single inch off its original location, or if there was a spot on the carpet left un-vacuumed, my guardians would throw objects at us: books, plates, remote controls, batteries—anything within arm's reach. On several occasions, my guardians emptied a dirty cat-litter box over our heads. We had to sit in cat feces and urine until they were satisfied that we were contrite. Then we had to clean the whole mess up. We got no dinner on those nights.

School became my getaway, my time away from their threats and obsessive castigation. During the walk home from school, Vannesa and I spent time examining the flowers growing by the side of the road. We took detours to play with a lizard that might be scurrying through the tall grasses leading to my guardians' house. But we had to be strategic; our guardians knew how long the walk was, and if we were observably late a harsh punishment would be meted out, one we couldn't escape. Every step was on a floor of eggshells; every move calculated in terms of how much pain I could avoid at any given moment. After two years under my guardians' custody, the first signs of post-traumatic stress syndrome and panic disorder began to develop. Alongside that was the belief—the proof—that life was unrelenting and unforgiving and the sense that I might never again find a home.

I didn't realize these would become my "truths"—beliefs that had taken root deep inside me—all before my fifteenth birthday. They would become my understanding of life itself. With a belief system so deeply intertwined with your perception of how things work, it's difficult to see anything else, and hence experience anything else.

Most of the time, however, we don't see what belief systems we operate under, nor where nor why they first arose—at least not the ones that developed from traumatic events we experienced as children, or the ones we quietly distill from patterns of events that may show up in our lives, out of our control. Instead, we tend to experience something trying and either obsess about it or attempt to "move on" from it by pushing it out of our minds. Neither of these opposite and justifiable reactions, two variations of the primal fight-or-flight reaction, bring healing. Both only serve to continue the patterning.

The first step of yoga, namely taking on the task of the witness, is what first allowed me to see what belief systems I held on to. It took several years just to learn to sit quietly with myself, then several more of sitting and observing to see that beneath the depression and anxiety that characterized my teens and early twenties was mistrust of life, and an underlying fear of death. Specifically, a fear of working so hard, struggling so much, and dying so young, like my parents. I came to realize I perceived both of my parents as never getting to enjoy the "fruits of their labor," and I feared the same destiny for myself. Would all my hard work and struggle be in vain? Deep inside, I could not see my own life past my parents', and that fearful belief kept me captive.

What I didn't see then is something that is clear to me today. The premise that my parents didn't live to enjoy the "fruits of their labor" rests on one flawed assumption: that the fruits of our labor are somewhere out there, in the future. When I look back now, I see pictures of my parents with my sister and me, and the joy on their faces is unmistakable. I reminisce about my father's vast library and his antique classical instruments. I recall fondly that Brazilian guitar, which he strummed with such zest. I look back on the paintings and drawings my mother created, and I see a life lived with passion. I see also Mami's work cleaning people's homes not as demeaning—as a child I sometimes struggled with feeling shame about Mami's profession—but as *she* saw it. Her business card used to say, "Adding a personal touch to your home," a promise she lived up to. Mami made art pieces for every person she worked for, and each one of those people came to see her as part of their family. Furthermore, I now see Mami's volunteer work as an art teacher as love for her daughters. I see all of it as her striving to teach us about strength, perseverance, and grace, all of which she modeled beautifully. The truth is I have no substantial proof that my parents didn't enjoy the short lives they lived. If anything, the evidence suggests the exact opposite. I have, in fact, the words of my mother that followed the statement of struggle I adopted— words that I ignored until recently. *It's worth it.*

The Work: Patterning and Restraint

By the time I moved to New York City, without any social, emotional, or financial support, I had cut off communication with any remaining family, with the exception of an occasional call to my sister. I carried deep resentment and bitterness, and believed I was better off alone. During my first few years in the city, I moved fourteen times. With every apartment, a situation arose where I found it impossible to settle. Whether it was financial, or roommates I couldn't bear, a flooding, or getting robbed, something always seemed to happen that would result in my breaking a lease. Moving within New York City is no easy task, and I found myself living out of boxes, packing up months or even weeks after I'd just finished unpacking. Each move intensified my anxiety, and I felt that my predicament was out of my control.

By this time in my journey, I had begun to practice witnessing, and was starting to awaken to the truth of my situation. But I still felt like a victim of circumstances. When I sat to observe, I noticed that the feelings associated with my constant moving were very familiar. I'd experienced them first after my father's death when we relocated from Colombia, during the time we had no place to call home—while sleeping in sleeping bags with my sister and mom, living out of a car, or in the rat-infested garage—and then again with the incessant trek from foster home to foster home after her death.

To understand yoga is to understand our patterns. Upon gaining clarity about my situation, I also noticed a big difference between the predicament of my early youth and my current situation. Then, I was a child, unable to take decisive action and under the care of my parents or other parties. Now, even though I didn't feel it, I had to know that it was through *my* decisions that I was choosing to re-create these traumas. It was not only very possible but even *likely* that I was creating circumstances that reflected my childhood wounding, even if they were painful and didn't serve me.

This was one of the first major truths I learned from witnessing: we re-create what we know, almost as though we are placing ourselves in the same situations to give ourselves the opportunity to outgrow that knowledge and choose differently. Most of the time, however, we're habituated and instead take on victimhood in light of the familiar pains that seem to return to haunt us. This is especially the case when, as it was for me, one believes that life is hard. If life weren't hard enough, then, so long as I held that belief, I would unconsciously ensure that it retained a certain degree of difficulty. This way my external world remained consistent with my internal one.

The Sanskrit word for this phenomenon is *saṁskāras*. *Saṁskāras* are the emotional patterns and impressions that take place within. After some time, these restrict our thoughts (and hence our actions) so they line up with what we already perceive to be true. When painful events affect us as children we may not have the tools necessary to deal with profound, heavy emotions like grief, anger, and displacement. We may not have lived long enough to understand that all things, including deep emotions, will pass. So, we create maladaptive strategies to cope with what's there, often resulting in withdrawing, ignoring the situation, or isolating ourselves. The more we utilize these strategies, the deeper their patterning will become; and the more we practice them, the better we get at them. The deeper the patterning, the more difficult it is to shift.

I like to refer jokingly to *saṁskāras* as little elves digging pathways in the brain. When a thought/behavior is established and repeated over and over, that neural pathway is physically deepened in the gray matter of our brain. We now recognize this phenomenon as neuroplasticity, one of the greatest discoveries of the twentieth century (found anywhere between twenty and twenty-five centuries *after* the *Sūtras* were written). In crude terms, neuroplasticity is the process by which the brain's neural pathways are altered because of environmental, physical, or behavioral changes. The process is complex, but for our purposes I'd like to highlight that it contradicts what people believed for ages: that we are born with a certain number of brain cells, and die with the same number; that we can't change the way our brain operates. Instead, we now know that the brain continues to alter its pathways as new information comes in. Although the process is nuanced, it's a theoretical parallel to yogic wisdom: We have the ability to change the patterns in the mind.[10]

Craving and Restraint

The mind and body tend to gravitate toward the path of least resistance; hence, the deeper the proverbial crevice of habit, the more likely we are to (inadvertently) choose that too-familiar route. Familiarity feels good, even if what we're familiar with causes pain. Addiction to behaviors works in this way. If a person one day decides to chew a stick of gum after dinner and rather enjoys it, and then decides to do it again and again, chewing gum after dinner becomes their normative way of being until it no longer feels like a choice is involved. The person just does it, unconsciously. The same can be said for anything, from cursing to pornography, from overeating to self-injury. With each of our addictions, a patterning and release (both emotional and chemical) occur from our engaging in the chosen activity.

It's no coincidence that the word *restraint* is used in the yogic conversation regarding yoga—the liberation from the suffering of our patterning. In fact, later in the yogic texts freedom is described as the state of non-thirst, non-craving.[11] Behind every addiction is a deep craving, a (perceived) thirst for the object we desire. The craving can be so strong that it often has the power to override other important values, including reason, empathy, and even love. In the clutches of craving, our behavior is often reactionary and without space; we may behave in ways that we know are not in our best interest, and even in ways that can hurt the people we love, despite our full awareness of the repercussions of our actions. That is how powerful craving can be. In effect, we feel torn up inside by a sense of separateness and continue the cycle of suffering. Unless we recognize the patterning and work our way out of it, the pattern becomes self-perpetuating and the habit becomes increasingly ingrained, so much so that it becomes entrenched into our most basic operating system.

Yogic wisdom suggests that when we look deeply at the nature of craving, we can find that our thirst is often not for the object we use to satiate ourselves with; what we crave is not cigarettes, food, or casual sex. Instead, these are Band-Aids we use at some point to cover over a deeper, unmet need within us. These maladaptive strategies fill us up until they no longer work, and so we come back to them again and again as momentary distractions from the craving's pull, which, in that moment, owns our consciousness. They help keep us away from a truth that might be scary to face, though deep inside we know they're not the answer.

The pull of craving and desire can be intense, physiologically speaking. Whether we find ourselves drawn to doughnuts, porn, or in my case the irresistible urge to pull my hair out, it is a bodily state of want. The more we temporarily satiate the object of that desire, the stronger the hold that object will have on us, and the deeper the pathways of *saṁskāras* in our neural wiring become.

It's helpful to recall how desire works in order to disentangle ourselves from it. When we examine a phenomenon, we create space between ourselves and the object we're observing. Within that space, choice abides. In the yogic deconstruction of desire, two important elements arise. First, desire originates from our senses. This, then, is our initial step out of conditioning. Although we may not have had much choice about what we were exposed to as children (what may have created that original sensation of lack), as autonomous adults we have choices. We can choose to shift the paradigm by changing the way we view our environment—from that which we are exposed to, to that which *we expose ourselves to*. Here is where yogic restraint comes into play.

Yogic restraint is not about controlling the mind to keep everything out. Restraint has both a soft and firm quality. Restraint entails taking responsibility for that which is around us—the raw materials from which we create our desires. If, for example, I am trying to give up refined sugar to improve my health, then one of the first things I must do is lessen my exposure to it, perhaps by emptying my kitchen cabinets and refrigerator of it. This is restraint. There is no problem that can be properly solved while we remain surrounded by the problem. To practice restraint is to simultaneously lessen the holding pattern by consciously restricting its availability. Restraint is then a very useful tool.

To use an example, say you decide to remove refined sugar from your diet and you practice restraint in your exposure by ridding your house of anything containing it. You ask for food in restaurants without the ingredient (when you realize that almost all restaurant food contains added sugar, you may decide to start preparing your own lunches to take to work). And you read all labels in the store to ensure that refined sugars stay out of your body.

At first, this task is painstakingly difficult; this period is, perhaps, the most challenging of all phases of releasing ourselves from the clutches of craving. Depending on the substance, you may experience headaches, lethargy, or mood swings. Withdrawal from caffeine, sugar, nicotine, and even gluten can result in some of these side effects. We may become frustrated at the realization that what we're avoiding seems suddenly to be *everywhere*. Everything has sugar in it; if we're quitting caffeine, Starbucks coffee houses seem to be on every corner. If we are distancing ourselves from pornography, every other website we click on has a pop-up advertisement of a sexual nature, calling our name. Even cleansing ourselves of toxic relationships or habitual patterns, such as negative self-talk, or healing OCDs like trichotillomania can have this effect. You feel off without that stimulus, and you find yourself noticing small things that remind you of that something or someone everywhere you look. This is when the contemplative yogic aspect can be so effective. During times of duress, coming into the body through techniques such as conscious breathing, accessing the body in present time, and tapping into the reality that this too will pass can be extremely helpful. (We will explore some of these techniques in the Workbook.)

As we progress down our path, even if we slip up occasionally, we may find that sugar's hold on us has relaxed a little bit. Instead of thinking about our craving every five minutes, a day will come when we realize, *Wow. I didn't think of sugar at all today.* Then, a couple weeks might go by where sugar is simply a passing thought, and those occasions when it comes into our field of awareness are when other people are eating something sweet around us. Still, we stay true to our progress, and, after a while, we notice in retrospect that even being around people eating sugar has stopped triggering the desire. So, on we continue, as the chain of craving loses hold, until the day comes where not only is the desire gone, but it doesn't even *sound* good to have sugar, and perhaps having some might make you feel a little bit sick.

This process could take months or even years, depending on how deeply embedded the patterning is, and my crude time-lapse version of the erosion of the craving and the rewriting of *saṁskāras* don't do justice to the challenge of the experience itself. Nonetheless, my point stands. Eventually, it *will* pass, and the relationship to sugar/caffeine/pornography and addictive tendencies as a whole will change as the observer—as you—change. This is simply our neural wiring; it just so happens that for the most part we are not taught how to operate it.

One drastic difference between the person desiring the sugar and the one who has overcome that desire is in the perceived lack. This is the second yogic point in regards to the nature of desire: You cannot have desire without a perceived lack, without a hole that seems to want to be filled.

The first layer in the work of restraint is this external one, which I have just described. However, there's more going on in this process on an internal level, which I find to be at least helpful (if not integral) to the process, and that is the "energetic" understanding of what is happening as we move toward nonattachment, which the *Sūtras* refer to as "the consciousness of self-mastery."[12]

Perceived lack is more than simply a desire for caffeine, sweets, or sex. It reflects a dearth of fundamental human needs: safety, security, acceptance, connection, trust, and love. The deeper, more contemplative work of yoga is to recognize that our deep patterns and sense of lack are a roadmap to something more—to areas in ourselves that may have gone neglected or may have suffered when we did not have the tools to heal them.

As we grow in our personal evolution, the work of yoga is to take responsibility for our healing and grow interested in our mindless patterning as a guide that can lead us to the gold: the underlying emptiness that has us reaching out, aching to be filled. Once we find what we're missing, we start rebuilding. It's this very study of our patterning that acts as a way out of it; the antidote for the ailment lies in the nature of the ailment itself. Once we dive in, we slowly make our way to the most fundamental truth of yoga: that we are already, and have always been, complete.

9

THE SEER AND THE OTHER

Depth psychologist Carl Jung said that everything that irritates us about other people can lead us back to an understanding about ourselves. In a sense, yoga is a self-centered philosophy and practice because one of its basic premises is that we are the conduits of our own experience; we see things on the outside as they exist for us internally.

Patañjali's fourth *sūtra* tells us that when we are not in the state of yoga, we assume the fluctuating mind-states.[13] This is to say that all the mumbo jumbo of the mind— the grocery and to-do lists, rambling thoughts we habitually get caught up in, and stories we are inclined to tell—becomes our reality. When we are caught up in the fluctuations of the mind, we identify with these things. We take them personally, and from there make decisions that further contribute to emphasizing and integrating that story into who we believe ourselves to be. In this chapter, I explore the relationship between our inner dialogue and our external world, the world where our relationships play out. Traditional commentaries on the *Sūtras* utilize a familiar metaphor: the metaphor of the still lake at night. My adaptation of it follows.

The Lake, the Other, and the Container

Imagine you are at the edge of a lake in the middle of a beautiful, quiet summer night. Nothing is moving, and it is tranquil and serene. As you look into the water you see your own reflection. The water is so still that you can even make out the details of your face, and the way your hair falls over your forehead. In the metaphor, the "you" that is looking into the lake is the Self (ātman, Soul, higher Self).

The lake is representative of the mind. When the mind is clear and at peace, we see ourselves as we truly are: joyful, creative, and at ease. The small disturbances seem to dissolve, and we can let things go and abide in the home of our expansive, bigger-picture Self. Say, however, that the wind blows and its gusts become stronger and stronger. The wind creates ripples and waves on the lake's surface. Your reflection becomes distorted, and the image is grossly skewed. If you take the ripples and waves personally, if you internalize and believe them, it might seem to you that your face actually *is* warped. It requires you to take a step back to realize that the distortion is occurring merely in the reflection, and that you, the witness, are unharmed by the winds.

The wind represents events—the ever-changing, occasionally intense and at other times milder circumstances that present themselves in our lives. The waves—the distortion in the water—is our "mind-stuff," the mental clutter and storm of reactivity that arise when the winds of change blow through our lives. When the mind is in constant commotion, our entire field of perception becomes distorted.

Events in our lives can create frenzy in our thoughts, shaking up the bottom of our lake, where the sands of our past may have lain still for years, or even decades. The degree to which our lake is disturbed is in direct proportion to the distortion of our self-image, our egoic (lower-case "s") self. Furthermore, the deeper we are conditioned to believe ourselves to be our egoic self, the more we lose sight of who we really are amid the winds of change, the more we associate with that discomfort, and the more that becomes our prevalent experience.

This metaphor extends further. As we look into the water, we not only see our own reflection but that of the rest of the world—the trees, the sky, the moon, and anything or anyone that may be in the background. When the lake is disturbed, when our mind is cluttered, our ability to see and connect with our Self isn't the only thing affected: everything else we see in the lake is affected. When our minds are colored by, say, an emotion like anger, the interpretation of what's around us will be similarly colored. Hence, to think that the judgments we hold toward ourselves are exclusively inward-pointing and don't change the way we encounter others, or to say that the judgments we make about others aren't related to how we feel about ourselves, is a fallacy. Our perception functions globally: the lens through which we see ourselves is the same as that through which we experience the Other.

A tremendous paradigm shift occurs when we see the Other. We question the nature of the self in relationship to the world. We have, as part of our human consciousness, a distinct sense of "self"—of "I am me"; the "me" feeling. This is, according to the sages, primarily just a feeling. When we reflect on our human experience, we come to realize that, truly, we do not know ourselves outside of the context of our environment: there has never been an isolated "you." In fact, since there was a "you," whether at conception, ensoulment (the moment that, in many traditions, the soul is believed to enter the body—often considered to be at conception or during quickening), or birth, you were encapsulated within an oceanic consciousness.

In the womb, you were part of something greater and could not survive without a mother. Even outside the womb, it takes months for infants to learn to distinguish their own hand as separate from anything else. Through the development of the human brain, along with learned experiences and the continual instillment of identity (e.g., your parents repeatedly calling you by your name), we learn that we are "singular." The *Sūtras* point out a critical truth: We are not separate from our context; we are not foreground to a background of Otherness. That layering happens only in our egoic aim for self-identification in contrast to what surrounds us. Although we may experience ourselves as primary, the reality is that our consciousness operates within an expanse of simultaneous activity. We are one thread in a big tapestry of ever-present consciousness that was here before we arrived and will exist long after we leave.

When we pull a single thread from a quilt, the patch from which it came is affected, and the fabric may shred. Every fragment of the tapestry matters, as it has its role in the creation of the whole. The judgments that we carry play a part in the larger space of consciousness that we contribute to both locally and globally. In the sphere of personal relationships, for example, it is said that in marriage you are only as happy as the less happy person. If you come home to a constantly dissatisfied partner, the chances of her or his unhappiness affecting your own mood are high. Said simply, we affect one another. The conditioned, autopilot response tends to be one of blame and fault-finding in the world. The yogic wisdom encourages us first to look within. Whether we are the grumpy one in the relationship (applicable to all relationships, romantic or otherwise), how we interpret and react to another's moods has something to tell us about ourselves. Chances are that we are not as open, conscious, and compassionate as often as we could be. Chances are that we are operating primarily from our self-centered stories.

* * *

The paradigm shift that yogic wisdom asks us to consider is that our notion of personal identity as singular is in many ways a grand (if not the grandest) illusion. Our existential situation is such that what feels like the foreground (ourselves) and the background (everything/everyone else) are not as separate as we might experience it through the ego; and that experience is largely conditioned. (This knowledge appears to be demonstrated by other, more communal, aboriginal societies, where the concept of the individual is downplayed, if not almost absent.) Instead, foreground and background are one, and how we experience it is a matter of focus, of where we choose to look. Our gaze, largely untrained, determines how we experience our background and ourselves; furthermore, the quality with which we experience one is the same as we experience the other. What we see in ourselves (whether we want to admit it or not) we see in the Other. What we judge in the Other is ultimately a judgment we hold about ourselves. This principle is the key to the wisdom at hand: The Other is ultimately a key to the Self.

To use a pragmatic example of how the principle of the Other in the lake plays out, imagine this: You're going to a friend's fancy birthday party and, on your way, you realize that you forgot to put on your dress shoes and don't have enough time to run home and grab them. You're already running late and you promised the host you'd be on time, so you decide to attend with inappropriate footwear—your beat-up sneakers. You may worry what people are going to think, if everybody will notice, and if people will judge your shoes and how you might reply to them, apologizing or explaining your situation. Once you arrive, the first thing you do is start looking at other people's shoes, and compare them with your own, judging both in the process.

Granted, the shoe example is tired, but it gets to the heart of the issue: We notice most in others the places where we have work to do. That's one reason why we occasionally interpret people so differently. Our experiences of others are intertwined with our own unresolved areas, and can manifest as anything from a judgment we jump to upon meeting someone new to an obsession with something someone does. Once again, yogic wisdom encourages us to take our relationships, from casual acquaintances to deep partnerships, as a roadmap to the Self. It encourages us to take a careful look at the attributes in others that may arouse something within us—discomfort, irritation, jealousy, etc.—and pair them with our experience of ourselves. In the end, any judgment toward the Other must first have an initial impetus within us. Could it be that the reason we're bothered by the way our coworker speaks is because she uses the same type of verbal crutches we had growing up for which we were teased? In the Workbook, we will dive into actual exercises that help us explore our shadow—exercises that will aid us in bringing light into these areas of unconsciousness. We will explore what to "do" there.

The Container

The second layer to the projection aspect of seeing ourselves in the Other is the concept of "the container." The truth of my Selfhood is that it is container-free. Alas, I am fallible and prone to human pettiness, and when I am operating from my pettiness the experience of myself becomes harnessed, tightened by the limits of my understanding—contained. The container allows us to hide from how things are (free and united); hence, the foibles in my understanding leave me feeling locked up, captive and separate, even though in actuality this isn't my truest nature.

When we are unaware of our expansive nature, we tend to live in identification with our thoughts and environment, which incarcerate our sense of self. It happens; it's okay, but we can learn to become aware of our tendency to contract, and mediate the contraction of our consciousness through tools that deepen our awareness and take us back to the greater truth. We know from both yogic wisdom and our own experiences that the smaller the container (the more intense the identification with a belief), the stronger the sense of isolation, pain, and discomfort.

Yoga is, and happens upon, the removal or enlargement of our personal container. In other words, yoga in action is the growth of our consciousness into its truest, freest form. This occurs when we realize that our inherent expansiveness is more real than the pettiness that keeps us locked up. It is a shift in our understanding.

Imagine taking a tablespoon of salt and dropping it in a cup of water, and then taking a drink. It's salty, right? But what happens if we add that same salt to a freshwater lake and taste it then? The salt disperses, and it's not so potent. In this metaphor, the water is our ego, the salt is the challenges we face, and the container in which the water is deposited is the self. When the container of the self is small, the ego becomes contracted and the salt in our lives will be experienced as saltier. Yoga is a mechanism by which we learn to enlarge the container of the self so that the ego expands and the salt dissipates. The ego as such is constantly expanding or contracting (mostly unconsciously), and through the process of yoga, we can learn to take ownership of our experience and re-expand when we notice a tightening—the very tightening that is at the center of our suffering. When the container of the self expands, allowing the ego to soften and open, our self-identity transforms. It moves from limitation toward limitlessness, and in this way, according to the ancient wisdom, it comes closer to the truth of who we ultimately are.

As we have learned from the *Sūtras*, the way in which we experience ourselves is inextricable from the way we experience others, and we know this on an intuitive, or even common-sense, level. That connection between self and others is the reason why if you're going to ask a friend a favor and you find out that they've had a terrible day, you might wait until they feel better to ask; because you know that if they are stressed, they may feel that your favor is an additional burden. Likewise, when our lake is clear and our container expanded, we experience ourselves—and hence other people—in a clear and open way. This is why, when we are at peace and someone in our lives behaves childishly, rather than blaming or associating that person with their actions (e.g., "they're a bad/selfish/angry person"), we are more likely to see that person beyond their behavior, and thus be more apt to forgive them. When we are in a space of clarity, we can more easily access compassion and say, "He's going through a hard time right now; that's why he has a short fuse today," without retaliating or taking their behavior personally.

When our container is full, we can't readily connect to others. Instead, we are likely caught up in protecting our fragile ego. In this state, we've lost our ability to be with what's here, and if left untended, we might even reach our breaking point.

It's worthwhile to note that in our culture we pay a lot of attention to physical cleanliness, but we don't pay the same attention to our mental, emotional, and spiritual hygiene. What if one morning you only put new clothing on top of yesterday's clothes? If this behavior continued for months, or even years, you'd not only be very uncomfortable, but the clothing would smell and rot.

This is what we tend to do with our emotional and mental laundry—we let it pile up. In times of extreme duress, when our container continues to fill with experiences that cause pain, we are less likely to behave from a place of openness and kindness toward others simply because the space to do so isn't available to us. Additionally, we may be more inclined to react to situations with blame, unable to take responsibility due to our sheer "fullness." In a very practical way, this causes strain on our relationships.

Through work within ourselves, our relationships with others can undergo a drastic metamorphosis. We can begin by learning to observe the ripples in our lake (our mental patterns and habits that lead to judgment of ourselves and others), and then use techniques that aid us in the calming of the water (such as those discussed in the Workbook). This creates the space we need to access peace and compassion for ourselves and, hence, for those around us. This is the process of waking up: moving from autopilot reactivity to a conscious response. Waking up begins with observation and is nurtured by our continually clearing our internal space so it might continue to grow. It is this process that results in freedom. The changes that transpire as a result of tending to our internal lake can't help but grow outward, and as a result, change the way we experience our lives.

The shift from automatic reaction because of an unconscious response and a full container to a conscious response where there is space and compassion begins with the self and can be a challenging undertaking. As we come closer to the realization that events as we perceive them and people as we understand them are largely that way because of our own perception of them—tainted by the stories we tell ourselves and the identities we attach to—we come closer to an understanding that we create our own experience. This radical shift demands radical responsibility for our internal world. If the lens we perceive ourselves through is the lens through which we perceive the world, and if the nature of our reality is infinitely interpretable, then we are left with the marvelous and massive responsibility of meaning-making. Meaning-making is an endeavor we take for granted and usually perform unconsciously.

Philosopher and teacher Alan Watts points out that one of the primary aims of the philosophies of South and East Asia is to challenge and ultimately change the perception of the self. It is within the self that the rest of the world gains meaning, and it is from this meaning that our actions and behavior are born. When we experience judgment, anger, or resentment toward others (either because of our own untended shadows or as a result of not clearing our container), the experience takes place *within us*. This is to say that there is nothing that can be projected that doesn't originate primarily within ourselves. One Buddhist proverb reminds us that holding anger is like having a hot coal in one's hands with the intention of throwing it at someone. We are always the ones who get burned first.

The path of yoga asks us to engage in a dynamic self-study as the catalyst for improving the world around us. We can't hope for a happy, healthy, and compassionate world if we don't cultivate those same principles within ourselves. This is our responsibility. Furthermore, the yogic path reminds us that the nature of our world is purely contextual. There is no isolated self outside of everything around us; all parts are united, the way a drop of water is both singular and simultaneously one and the same as the ocean itself. It is by tending to the ripples in our lake, clearing the waters of our mind, and expanding the capacity of our selfhood that we can become translucent and finally see ourselves, and each other, clearly.

I didn't have the guts to test my guardians' boundaries. I was too afraid of them. But Vannesa wasn't. At fifteen, my little sister was fiercer than I could ever be. She stood up for herself often, and on several occasions was pushed against the wall and choked almost to the point of losing consciousness. She told me it was worth it. When Vannesa told Phillip, her high school boyfriend, that he could stay with us while our guardians, Ron and Jenna, were out of town for the day, I opposed it immediately.

"No way. You're crazy," I said.

"Why? What are they going to do that they haven't already done?"

"They'll kill us." I wasn't sure if I meant that only figuratively.

"But he has nowhere to go," Vannesa said. Phillip sat on the porch, icing a black eye, his shirt caked with blood. Like us, Phillip was also a foster child. He was the son of a crack-addicted mother and had been churned through the foster-care system like we had been. His guardian had a habit of beating him up when he didn't behave, which was often.

"I don't think so," I said.

"Please? It's not like we're going to do anything bad. We'll just hang out in the back room."

I looked out at Phillip through the window.

"Look," Vannesa pressed on, "their daughter used to bring guys over all the time. And they stayed the night and her parents never cared. Why would they care if I have Phillip over? I mean, how bad could it be?"

She was right. At least we had that going for us. If we got caught, we could pull the hypocrisy card.

"Fine. Go to the back room. But he has to be out before Ron and Jenna get home."

"Thank you, thank you, thank you, thank you, thank you!" Vannesa chanted as she ran outside to get Phillip. When he came in, he gave me a hug: "Thanks, sister." I nodded. He liked to call me *sister* from time to time, to emphasize our unity in the struggle of foster-hood. His face looked tired and beat-up—not just from his guardian's punches, but from life itself.

It was a sunny Saturday morning, and normally Vannesa and I would be on our knees with toothbrushes cleaning toilets until dinner. Today, however, the Johnsons decided they wanted to go on an outing beyond the limits of our little 2,500-person town. Oakdale was nestled in the California Sierras where the air was fresh, the trees were hefty and tall, and Main Street was decorated with signs for the next rodeo. So we had the house to ourselves, and nothing sounded better than curling up on my bed with a book. Then I dozed off.

"Hello?!" I heard as a door slammed. I looked at the clock on my nightstand: 3:45 P.M. They weren't supposed to be back until nightfall. It took half a second for the severity of the situation to fully hit me. Phillip was still here. I prayed anyway: *God, if you exist, please, please, please let Phillip have gone home.*

"Helloooooo!" Ron called again, not so much as a greeting, but more of a demand. I heard the footsteps approach my room. *Stall him,* I thought.

"Hi, Ron!" I yelled, in an attempt to warn my sister in the room adjacent to mine.

"Where's your sister?" he demanded.

"I fell asleep reading," I replied, avoiding his question.

"Where's Jenna?" *Shit, shit, shit. He knows.*

"She's at the neighbor's," I said, as Ron started to walk away from my room and began to look around.

I shot up out of bed. "How was shopping?" I asked.

"Fine. Why is the door to the back room closed?" Ron asked, as he walked farther down the hallway. "Vannesa?!" he demanded. "Vannesa?!" I heard scrambling.

Shit. There is no god. He's still here. Phillip is still here.

"One minute," Vannesa called, a slight tremble in her voice.

"Why the fuck do you need a minute?!" he yelled back, going for the doorknob. It was locked. That was not allowed. "Why the fuck is this door locked?!" he demanded, outraged.

More scrambling.

"I'm . . . I'm changing," she replied.

"Open this goddamned door right now!" he screamed.

I was paralyzed, my feet like anvils, my head spinning. Ron pounded his fists on the door, which shook against his weight. Finally, Vannesa unlocked the door, and it swung open with the force of Ron's body, hitting the wall behind it.

"I was changing," she said. No Phillip.

"Something isn't right here," he said.

Oh God, no! Please no. If there is a god, please don't let him find Phillip. I knew exactly where she'd hidden him. Ron stepped into the room, looking around. He went straight for the closet door. My heart stopped.

"You fucking little whore!" Ron yelled, as Phillip stumbled out of the closet. Phillip tried to make a run for it but didn't manage to escape Ron's fist. Blood flew and hit the door. "I'm going to kill all of you!" Ron yelled, his eyes wide and filled with rage. As Phillip recovered from the punch, he fled down the hallway and out the back door while Ron raced to his closet to retrieve his shotgun. This gave Phillip enough time to get a head start down the driveway, but Ron was not far behind him, screaming, "My bullets are faster than you, you little shit!"

Vannesa had fainted after Ron hit Phillip, drops of his blood splattered on her face. She lay unconscious on the floor until I could finally move and pick her up. Her face was ashen. Ron stormed back into the house. Phillip had gotten away. Vannesa began to come to, stirring softly. Suddenly, Ron appeared in the doorway, shotgun in hand. He was furious. Large red veins bulged from his hands and forehead. He pointed the gun at us. "Whose idea was this!?" he demanded. I felt a warm trickle on my lap and down my leg; Vannesa had wet herself. Her eyes rolled back, she went limp again, and I caught her.

"I said, whose idea was this?" Ron repeated.

"It was mine," I lied. "Phillip got beat up and had nowhere to go."

"I don't give a shit. He probably deserved it."

"Jessica," I said, stuttering, "Jessica had lots of boys over and she didn't get in trouble. That was for fun and this was to help Phillip."

"You two are not Jessica. Jessica is my daughter, and she can do as she pleases in her own house. This is *not* your house, you dirty whores. We take you in and this is how you repay us?" he exclaimed, the gun still in our faces.

Just kill us, I thought and closed my eyes. *Just end this misery right now. I don't want to live in fear anymore.* I opened my eyes and looked straight down the eye of the barrel. I imagined the bullet coming at me in slow motion, pictured it puncturing my forehead, straight into my brain. Then I looked up at him.

"Pack your pathetic sister's shit," Ron said. "I'm done taking care of kids that aren't mine. Especially a bitch like this one." He pushed Vannesa with the wrong end of the rifle. Vannesa had regained consciousness but was still pale and could barely move. I was shaking and thought I might vomit. Ron put the gun down and took it back to his room. "I'll be waiting in the car," he said as he walked out. I changed my little sister's soiled clothes and packed a bag for her, even though I had no idea where he was taking her.

Vannesa and I sat in the back seat of Ron's car holding hands, our little fingers intertwined as he drove west and intermittently shouted profanities at us. Rush Limbaugh's voice droned on in the background. At stoplights, Ron would reach back to punch my sister in the legs, or wherever he could reach. I tried stopping him to no avail. This is how my sister and I were separated, only two years after Mami's death.

When our container is full, our reactions take over. The intensity of the reactions is directly proportional to the amount of cleanup that needs to be done; to how much has been stored inside that we haven't taken responsibility for, that we haven't looked at, shed light on, or cleaned out. No trespass justifies pointing a gun at a child, or relating to a child with the degree of violence my sister and I experienced at the hands of our guardians. I know this now, as an adult.

Healing doesn't happen in linear time. One only needs a cursory understanding of quantum physics to realize that time, as we experience it, is illusory, or not something strictly linear. In fact, I'd say that sometimes healing requires a sort of time travel, revisiting old hurt to reframe it in a new context: the safety of the present moment. With a new understanding of what happens when our container is full, and with the knowledge that we are the keepers and healers of our own wounds, it's possible to revisit our past and restructure our experience through the lens of compassion. In so doing, we heal ourselves where we are now.

When I look at my experience with my guardians through the lens of my pain and recall the abuse and the fear they instilled, and when I look at the ways in which their mistreatment created even more maladaptive coping mechanisms within me, old conditioned feelings of sadness, fear, and anger can easily arise. Yet, when I look at the past through the work of yoga, and in this case, the work of the Other, I know for a fact that for a person to project that much pain onto someone else, especially a defenseless child, *they* must be undergoing an enormous amount of suffering. When a person misuses their power and dominates the powerless, it's because they feel that way within themselves—they are holding the hot coal. Suffering begets suffering. If I can, even for a moment, consider that some people are not exposed to the tools of self-analysis and the work of the inner self, then I can feel compassion for their experience. Although this in no way justifies their actions, I can feel sympathy for the degree of toxicity that must be present inside them for them to react so violently, to lack all control of automatic reactions, to be a prisoner to those emotions, and to ruin valuable relationships in the process.

In the end, I was able to escape that abusive household, but to this day I'm not sure if my guardians were able to escape the prison within themselves. For this, I feel compassion. In the space that compassion creates, the pain they caused me lessens, because it's not about me anymore—it stops feeling so personal. That doesn't excuse abusive behavior, nor does it make the other party any less responsible. However, it does shift *my* perspective, and hence the quality of, and my relationship with, my own pain.

I wouldn't have been able to arrive at that space without entering the doorway of the yogic understanding of the Other. Through obtaining this new lens, I gained insight into another's plight, and changed my automatic response. I feel certain that had my guardians had access and chosen to undertake this type of work within themselves, I would never have found myself, sixteen years old, holding my trembling sister, and looking down the barrel of a gun.

10
MY PERSONAL HELL

I first had the idea to cut myself a few months after Mami passed. I was fourteen. I don't know where the seed of that thought originated, but suddenly it made sense that I should try it. While my guardian was making dinner one night, I procured an X-Acto knife from her sewing kit, went into the bathroom, and locked the door. I retrieved a brown bottle of peroxide from under the sink and a cotton swab from one of the drawers. As I sat next to the bathtub on the floor, I dabbed peroxide on a portion of my leg near my ankle (where a sock would easily conceal it), and pressed the thin and shiny edge against my skin.

I did it softly at first, as though testing the temperature of water close to the boiling point. I applied a little pressure, and then a little more, until the skin gave in and a single crimson stream emerged. Transfixed, I watched as the blood trickled out of the cut. It was almost graceful, the way everything seemed to stand still for that instant, while a silky river flowed over my cinnamon skin. For that moment, the noise in my head quieted and I could breathe.

Although I couldn't quite put my finger on why it was "wrong" to cut myself, I knew it wasn't an activity I should be openly engaging in. It felt forbidden. So I promised myself I would stay away from the blade and tucked the incident away in the back of my mind.

Years later, the winter that I fell apart in New York City, I opened Pandora's box. On my way home from class, I stopped at a little hardware store a few blocks from the L train and bought the same kind of knife. I went to the bodega a block from my building and purchased a small bottle of peroxide. When I got home, I reenacted the scene from my youth and made a single cut on my arm. It was an instant high—the high of no thoughts—followed by profound guilt, the knowledge that it wasn't quite right. I promised myself again that I wouldn't use the blade, buried it in my sock drawer, and slammed it shut.

It felt as though the heaviness in my heart gained another pound with each passing day. I wanted nothing more than to alleviate that weight, and so my thoughts returned to cutting. Once you've felt an instant of relief from a relentless pain, you can't pretend you don't want that relief again. After being in a ruthless civil war within yourself, once you've found a serenity that resembles sitting on a mountain ledge overlooking a vast horizon, you can't pretend you don't want that peace again. In fact, it's all you want. So, I broke my promise. I opened the sock drawer.

The itch to cut grew more intense, until it became difficult to ignore. Each time I cut, the craving for more cuts deepened, as did the cuts themselves. As is the nature of addiction, what had once satiated me was soon no longer enough to generate the same relief, to keep the voices, memories, and anxiety away. I needed more marks, more blood, more catharsis. My cutting sessions evolved. First, they became weekly, and before long, I was cutting every other day, until I began to carry an X-Acto knife, cotton swabs, and a small bottle of peroxide with me in my book bag everywhere I went. Between classes I'd go into the bathroom, find the largest stall, and set up my cutting station. It became a routine, a fix, like smoking a cigarette after a meal, and just as normalized and justified in my head.

It was also a ritual, and at the time seemed almost sacred and beautiful. I arranged my tools always in the same alignment and measured my cuts with precision, lining them up one next to the other. When I cut at home, I lit candles and incense and sat on my bedroom floor. Everything was calculated. My ritual no longer necessitated tears, nor was it a last resort; if anything, it felt as though it was just a part of my self-care routine, like brushing my teeth or moisturizing my skin. Some girls got manicures; I cut myself.

Cutting always provided a reprieve from the suffering—a brief moment of stillness. Yet the memories, anxiety, and fear inevitably returned. Soon, my calves, thighs, abdomen, arms, ankles, and hips were covered with small incisions, all neatly arrayed like soldiers in battle formation. To this day, sixty-seven tiny scars cover the soft inside of my left arm alone; I never counted the rest, but there must be hundreds all over my body—hundreds of instances when the only way I knew how to deal with the hurt inside me was to embody it in my flesh, and voice its pain through blood.

My cutting eventually led to my hospitalization. By this time, my internal demons had become impossible to ignore. My head was covered in bald spots that I'd hide with a beanie, and my eyelashes and eyebrows were mostly gone. I'd lost over twenty pounds, hovering somewhere around eighty to ninety pounds, and unable to remember the last time I ate or cared to eat. Throughout, I was blind to the connection between my increasing need to cut, my insomnia, my panic attacks, and the PTSD symptoms that were re-emerging and intensifying. In my bed in Brooklyn, I'd lay awake unable and afraid to sleep—afraid to be thrown into a dream where I saw my father's head-on collision, or watched my mother die again, or relived the precarious years after her passing, where nothing was safe. I tried to run away from my memories by diving into graduate work, and spent countless nights at the library in an effort to avoid sleep.

In the quiet hours, the memories found me again—images of my parents alive and dead, and of foster care. The abuse my sister and I suffered in foster care was often physical, but it was primarily mental—and this was perhaps the worst aspect of all. The body is wondrous in its ability to mend itself after a physical injury has been inflicted. Mental wounds are a bit different. They are subtle and treacherous, like hidden landmines that undermine your defenses and can explode at any time.

Our guardians made Vannesa and me feel like outcasts. We weren't invited on family trips or included in family photos. When they were drunk or in a fit of rage, our guardians liked to berate one of us in front of the other, to see how many insults it would take to make the other break. When one of us broke, we'd be punished. It was always worse to be the sister who watched the other get humiliated. On the receiving end, I learned tricks to keep the insults and intimidation from getting to me: I counted numbers; I listed colors; I said Hail Marys over and over, praying for an intervention.

But it's different to see the person you love most and the last family member you have left in this world be hurt right in front of you. Still, we stayed quiet. We knew too well what doing otherwise would cost us—no food, more cleaning, their hands around one of our necks, threats of "knuckle sandwiches," and a big, white, wrinkly fist waving in front of our noses. Or the threat that they would separate us and send one of us away to another country, make sure we'd never know of the other again. But it wasn't the screaming, the blaming, or the intimidation that was the worst of it. The worst of all the punishments was a man named Manuel.

✳ ✳ ✳

Manuel was tall and dark, with the blackest hair I'd ever seen. He had a gap between his two front teeth. He'd been a friend of the family for years, and was especially fond of my mother. By "fond of," I mean he'd been infatuated with her for years. They dated for some time, but then she decided to leave the relationship for reasons I'll never know. After her death, Manuel would come to visit us, and on several nights he stayed over in the guest room. If I'd misbehaved somehow, the greatest punishment I faced was being made to share a bed with Manuel. There was nothing more terrifying than that bed, with that middle-aged man, in a room where he kept a red night-light on. Before he turned out the light, he liked to take his clothes off slowly. When his shirt came off, I cried. When his pants came off, my body shook in fear and my chest heaved. He seemed to enjoy the whole process. Once the night-light came on, the shadow of his undressed body lingered on the ceiling, dancing over my body's shadow all night. This was the Manuel punishment: sexual assault as castigation for not having cleaned properly, or for talking back—having my first sexual encounters be ripe with fear and non-consent; having my introduction to healthy sexuality stolen from me by this man, with the approval of the people who were granted legal guardianship over me.

On days he stayed the night, Manuel liked to drive Vannesa and me to school the following morning. He would drop us off by the school buses and park his shoddy, silver 1992 Buick a block away from the main building—far enough away where it wasn't obvious, but close enough to keep watch over us. During recess and lunch, I could see Manuel sitting in his car, trying to make me out from the crowd of teenagers. When he found me, I could feel his gaze burning into me. He wanted me to know he wasn't going anywhere; he wanted to remind me that I'd probably share a bed with him that same night.

I knew that after school was over, Manuel would drive back near the school buses, waiting to pick us up. I dreaded being in that car with him, where no excuse I made to sit in the back seat mattered. I'd inevitably end up in the front, his hand working its way up my thigh. If he was in a particular mood, he'd take the back roads and park the car somewhere behind a field, where we would not be easily spotted. He'd grab my face with his massive hands and press his ashtray mouth onto mine. I fantasized about biting his filthy tongue, ripping it right out from its root. But instead, I dug my nails into the car seat, tears streaming down my face, praying for it to be over. Vannesa had to sit in the back seat and look away, knowing neither one of us had any power; knowing that if we ever told anyone, they would separate us, even deport us—a fate that felt scarier than any of the things Manuel could do.

I was repeatedly threatened and sexually assaulted from the age of fourteen until my eighteenth birthday, when I was no longer legally bound to foster care. The day after I turned eighteen, I waited until my guardians were at work and skipped school to pack my things in plastic bags. I left without even a goodbye note. That was the last I saw of them for nearly a decade.

Back in New York, years later, I hadn't left behind what Manuel had done to me or the angst that still lingered in my body. Flashbacks from the abuse and assault haunted me for years. I still occasionally jolt awake screaming from a nightmare of his hands on my teenage body. He was the first male ever to kiss me or touch me in a sexual way, filling me with dread and revulsion. In these dreams, I feel suffocated and trapped. He's back, and I can again feel his hot breath on the nape of my neck, his stubble scratching my face. One of his huge hands is holding me down while the other is making its way up my thigh, and the stench of fresh bleach and cat litter permeates the air, making it hard to breathe.

"If you tell anyone," he'd whisper, "I'll kill your sister."

At the onset of our teenage years, when identity is a budding, delicate, and tenuous thing, distresses like these can create deep crevices in the foundation of who we are. My profound solitude in New York City forced me to come face-to-face with all those ghosts I'd shoved inside the closet of my consciousness. I know why I chose to ignore them: dealing with them meant having to acknowledge they happened in the first place, and reliving the pain was unbearable.

I'd lie awake night after night, caught in my personal hell, praying to my parents, searching for respite. Although I knew my parents didn't want to die, I was mad at them for doing so. I was angry at them for not leaving us any clues, directions, or advice for how to live our lives without them or how to deal with the pain. Papi had died in the car crash. It was unforeseen. But Mami, it seemed like she knew better, even though she only lived a few months after her diagnosis.

At night, I wrote endless letters to Mami. *Why couldn't you write me directions, tell me what to do, how to take care of Vannesa, how to take care of myself?* If she knew she was leaving, dying, then why not give us a few words of wisdom? I'd press the pen hard into the paper, almost ripping it. Fear and grief were like hot wax, burning then hardening. I'd find a pause—the moment when it became clear that there was nothing to be done; that perhaps she wasn't even there and couldn't hear me.

What is there, then, behind the silence, behind the realization that your mother is dead, that dead means *forever*, and that your father is with her: that it's been almost a decade since you've seen them both? What's beyond the realization that your children will never get to meet their grandparents, taste their grandmother's cooking, or hear their grandfather's Colombian folk melodies rising from his acoustic guitar? There is a gap. Space. Silence, and nothing else. I hated Mami for her dead, stupid silence, and I hated her for leaving us stranded, up to chance, up to pure faith. I hated her for trusting that we would survive.

Overwhelmed, and without a single tool at my disposal, I used the best and most cathartic ways I knew: pulling, starving, cutting. I opened a door to the wounds I had not yet healed, which had festered through my teenage years and now, in my early twenties, could no longer be denied.

From my room in New York, I called my sister, who remained in California. I told her I was having trouble sleeping, that days were melding into nights, and that I couldn't keep track of what was what. I told her that when I closed my eyes I had flashbacks of Mami dying in our arms, of the tubes that came out of her belly. I told her about the nightmares of being back with Manuel. My sister simply listened. I remember asking, "Vannesa, am I crazy?" to which she replied, with a gentle shakiness in her voice that I recognized as tears, "I don't know."

A few weeks later, a friend whom I'd known from college came to visit, and in a moment of carelessness I took off my sweatshirt and he caught a glimpse of my arms. From the outside, my friend had seen what I was blind to—a profound deterioration of my well-being. In many ways, I was unrecognizable.

I confided to my friend that I was overwhelmed by sadness and needed to "get away" for a while. I did as I planned, and sequestered myself, disconnected my phone, and hibernated until a date that I dreaded: October 26, the fifteenth anniversary of my father's passing. How was it, I wondered, that I once had everything and now felt so alienated? That night, after several days without contact with anyone, I sat in my room and began the cutting. This time I didn't stop after three, four, or five cuts. I didn't stop after twenty or thirty. I didn't stop after sixty. I didn't want to stop, or perhaps didn't know how to. Cut after cut after cut, deeper and deeper, I worked my way down to my wrists.

In the ambulance, the falling rain and the flashing lights blended into a glow. My arm was bandaged in the emergency room of Woodhull Hospital in the heart of Brooklyn. I was transferred from one hospital to another until I was admitted to Bellevue Psychiatric. I weighed a mere eighty-four pounds and was covered in gashes. I was diagnosed with severe depression, PTSD, panic disorder, OCD, self-injury, anorexia, and attempted suicide.

It must have been the tone in my *goodbye* that let my friend know that something was wrong. Today, I think often about the courage it took for him to make that 911 call. I think about how different my life might have been—or if I would have had any life at all—had he not trusted his intuition and made a very difficult decision that, at the time, felt to me like a betrayal. This incident speaks volumes to one of the primary truths of life that yoga reveals for us: our inherent connectedness, the fact that we are here together, and that we simply cannot heal in a vacuum.

11

THE SHIFT FROM
SELF TO SELF

Personal Pain

The range and depth of human experience is astonishing. The possible darkness can be overwhelming. Shadows can haunt us for years (even decades), and can appear at unexpected moments, triggered by even the most inconspicuous and benign life events. At the other end of the spectrum, the joy and peace available to us in the space of light can dazzle us with their brightness and serenity, healing even our darkest places. In between lies an almost endless variety of moods and emotions we all undergo regardless of the circumstances of our lives—from grief to delight, exhaustion to satisfaction. They are all part of the human condition.

For many of us, emotional states are habitual or unconscious; and for a certain group of us, they can be downright oppressive. Some of us, often considered the "highly sensitive," have emotions that can shift so wildly that they seem to control our entire experience of life, and others still appear to be genetically predisposed to depressive disorders,[14] for which other treatments can prove extremely useful, even necessary. That said, the principles of yoga provide extraordinary healing tools, both on their own and as a complement to other healing modalities. The yogic path is one of creating awareness in order to move from our emotions controlling us to choosing our experience and learning to intentionally create meaning in our lives.

The impetus for writing this book was my own complicated and long-term relationship with darker and more toxic emotions, and with my constant, and many times debilitating, struggle to fight against them. I have a vivid memory of myself as a young child crying in my mother's lap after a trip home from an orphanage my parents volunteered at on the outskirts of Bogotá. I'd asked my mom why the children had no families and how they could live in such poverty. She replied that life doesn't always seem fair and there were people in truly dire situations. It felt incomprehensible to me that such sadness could exist.

I remember how Mami consoled me as she stroked my head. She placed her hand on my chin and lifted it toward her: "Tatiana," she said, "you need to learn to strengthen your little heart or else life is going to be very difficult for you." My mother's words stayed with me, and they echo in my head when I feel waves of emotion threatening to throw me off-balance. My inherently sensitive disposition made my ensuing trauma that much harder on my mental, emotional, and spiritual well-being. Yet ultimately, this same sensitivity has led me on a healing journey through the yogic thought I'm presenting here—one that, after years of work and honing, has become one of my most valuable tools.

Puruṣa and Prakṛti

Yogic philosophy identifies two planes of consciousness: *puruṣa* and *prakṛti*. *Puruṣa* is pure, unadulterated, unmanifest consciousness and awareness; *prakṛti* is often translated as nature or movement. The manifest world is made of *prakṛti*—everything we experience through sense perception, all of nature, as well as what we experience in the mind, and the fluctuation of thought. In other words, the nature of nature is movement and change; anything that has movement is *prakṛti*, and everything in the manifest world changes.

Puruṣa, on the other hand, is unchanging. Because it is immaterial, it cannot be perceived or known directly through the senses. Yet, we still experience *puruṣa*, because we experience consciousness. *Puruṣa* is the consciousness underlying all things, and within the human experience, *puruṣa* is our quintessential Self, often referred to as the watcher, the soul, the highest Self.

As we've established, suffering from the yogic standpoint is primarily caused by a non-seeing, or a misidentification with what we are not, in the highest sense: namely, *prakṛti*. Because we are so driven by our senses, and everything that our senses perceive is *prakṛti*, it's easy to mistake our identity with *prakṛti*, that is, with the changing attributes of our selfhood—our careers, our belongings, our social status.

When constructs fall apart (as they most often will, because that is their nature), then we suffer. The process of healing through yoga comes about by recognizing our misidentifications and shifting them so we come to realize, to remember, our truest self: the unchanging awareness underlying all beingness—*puruṣa*.

This identification isn't just a philosophical quandary; it's relevant to our ordinary lives. The root of our identification underlies our behavior, and how we make our way through the day. When we believe that we *are* our careers or the car we drive, our actions in the world come from a segregated place. Conversely, when we are seated in a deep understanding of our truest nature, our behavior will arise out of wholesomeness; it is integrated, unified. This is why the *Sūtras* remind us that part of the path is a constant recalling of who we are. Because we are creatures of habit, the more we root ourselves in our understanding of *puruṣa*, the more we behave wholesomely, and the more this integrated behavior heals our perception of the segregated self, within which all suffering resides.

Shift from self to Self

Emotional pain, disconnectedness, *avidyā* (non-seeing), and illusion all live in the egoic version of the self that is attached to the *prakṛti* or changing states of the world. This version of the self is time-bound, and is often a precarious, attention-seeking, needy, and injured part of us that has the propensity to act from the underlying premise or experience of separation, often because of events that instilled a deep sense of loss, isolation, and fear.

Although emotional pains are very real, they are not the highest truth. Incidents like betrayal, loss, death, and abuse have a way of lingering, especially because the victim will often become hyperalert and take special precautions to prevent these types of occurrences from happening again. Unfortunately, as we've seen, it's likely (and painfully ironic) that our painstaking efforts to assure that whatever harm we have endured does not repeat itself are often the same behaviors that perpetuate the re-traumatization in our lives.

Take, for instance, a person who's been deeply betrayed by his partner. Swearing that he'll not repeat the mistakes of his past, he moves on to a different relationship with open eyes, suspiciously checking up on his new partner's behavior, scanning for signs of betrayal. He checks her phone when she's not in the room and looks through her emails when she leaves her computer open. Thus, the new partner, who may be perfectly loyal, feels insulted or hurt, resulting in a loss of trust. The "cautious" behavior taken to prevent betrayal only serves to create distance in his new relationship.

When we live in pain, we exist within the contracted and separated ego; again, think of the small cup filled with salt. In this place, the egoic self is in constant need of reassurance; it is ruled by lack, unconsciousness, resistance, separation, and fear, and has attachments to these. We can sense this truth for ourselves if we take a moment to examine our bodily sensations. Scanning the body, we gain insight into the state of the mind. When the mind operates from a place of separation and fear, the body reacts by feeling tight, stressed, rushed, overly watchful, and compacted. In this state, our thoughts often run on a singular track and are based on fleeting events—not the underlying truth behind all events—and we can become stuck.

Buddhist thought offers the Four Noble Truths, the first of which is that so long as we are embodied, we will suffer; this is simply the lot we come into the world with. Tragedy and loss are real and unavoidable aspects of our human experience, but the quality and the length of that suffering is up to us. When we (often unwillingly) per-petuate our internal suffering, the external world catches up to our expectations. Our fears become self-fulfilling prophecies. This is why so many people have dated "the same person" in fifteen different bodies; why we cycle over and over again, re-creating our worst nightmares. This wheel of patterns will continue and the lessons will be repeated until we choose to learn and grow from them. It's not until we examine and learn to identify our patterns and wholeheartedly ask ourselves, *What is going on here right now?* that we can shift our experience and change the quality of our lives.

In contrast to the egoic small self, the Conscious Self (our realization of *puruṣa*) is satiated. Unlike the egoic self, the Conscious Self is the aspect of our being attuned to our inherent connectedness. It behaves from the premise of compassion, peace, trust, and love. The distinction between self and Self simply serves to highlight that the Conscious Self is expansive, operates from a higher frequency, and isn't attached to outcomes; it isn't identifying itself with anything external. The Conscious Self abides in a space of allowance and love because it doesn't cling, push away, expect, or wish things were different.

The yogic paradigm begins with the basic premise that yoga—a state of recognized union and hence acceptance, freedom, and love for what is—is our truest state. The third *sūtra* tells us that in yoga, "the Seer abides in his own true nature."[15] In yoga, we fully embody the highest version of ourselves, and we can experience others in that same way. The pettiness of the contracted and attached ego falls away, making room for a greater, more open mind and heart. This openness creates a state of absolute compassion and connection. When we aren't operating with this openness, we tend to get caught up in our stories, our thoughts, our past or our future.[16] We cling to these things and build our identity around them. And we suffer.

The underlying premise of yoga is that healing occurs when we create a shift from isolation to union, which is to say, when we awaken to the reality that we are always already united. Our mission, should we choose to accept it, is to learn to identify that which feels segregated within us and merge it with where we are now, with the moment at hand. This is how we move into the completeness of who we truly are, and recognize that we have been complete all along. Our shift from self to Self, then, is our return home, to the truth of our present hearts.

Compassion
peace
trust
love

12

ILLUMINATING
THE DARKNESS

In ancient shamanic paradigms, everything, including non-sentient objects, has life. Such a worldview isn't so far-fetched when we remember that all things (you, me, this computer I'm typing on, the book you're holding) is made of the same "stuff." Particles vibrate at different frequencies to create an illusion of separate objects, but at the sub-atomic level, the boundaries are not so distinct. In shamanic paradigms, everything, animate or inanimate, whether it has a physical or non-physical composition, lives, moves, and vibrates.

Consider for a moment a thought experiment. Take the premise that everything lives and has the most basic sentience, in that in its aliveness its function is to express itself as the most authentic version of itself. Bring to mind that moment of blissful yogic union that occurs when you engage fully with the present, embedded in an activity that fulfills you wholeheartedly. In this space, you are seen and recognized, if by none other than yourself. This is the truest expression of you at your best. Shamanic wisdom asks: What if everything longed to express itself that way? What if everything, no matter the object or degree of perceived sentience, yearned to be seen for what it really is? What if emotions, for example, were personified—spirits of pure expression—and all they wanted in order to be released was simply to be acknowledged?

When emotions live deep within the shadows of unconsciousness, they are not seen, heard, acknowledged, or expressed. It might be helpful, as we engage in our yogic exploration of our experience, to consider, or at least momentarily imagine, that when personified, emotions perform the definition of their function: they emote. If we can step away from our identification with our emotions to create space between us and the emotion as such, we can imagine that emotions aren't us, nor are they ours to keep. What if emotions were their own transient entities and we were a vessel for their expression, a tool for them to channel and pass through? If we can momentarily imagine an emotion as its own "being," it no longer owns us, nor do we own it; we are not intrinsic to the emotion, and it is not intrinsic to us.

Research indicates that emotions, when left on their own, last approximately ninety seconds.[17] Yet, our experience seems to tell a different story. In graduate school, I remember reading a case study in a book on existential therapy in which a woman who'd had a brief romantic affair with a man was in therapy twenty years later, still caught in the pain of that lost love. This story resonated with me because I saw myself in it; I feared I'd become like that woman, because I knew my capacity to hold on to pain was just as strong as hers.

When we identify with an emotion, relive it, and obsess over it repeatedly, its lifespan can last years because that grasping is linked with identification. We believe and behave as though the pain is part of who we are, essential to our identity. In the grasping is both a misidentification with the emotion and an inability to let it express itself fully as something other than us, and thereby release it (we cannot release something we believe to be central to ourselves). Playing with deep emotions without consciousness is engaging in a dangerous game of entanglement. Imagine the internal shift we could undergo if we adopted a different perspective to our inner mud!

Much of our darkness remains unidentified. Without a name or clear constitution, it exists without proper acknowledgment. The darkness can exist in different ways in our emotional body: sadness, anger, fear, or simply unrecognized, malaise—that familiar feeling of stuckness. Conscious observation is the light of understanding. To sit with the intention of observing emotion as it transpires and learn to simply name and identify what we see creates a powerful space between us and what lies within us. In this space, we loosen the grip of attachment and misidentification. We learn that we can only really observe what isn't intrinsically us. The power of creating space to observe emotion and identify its expression without attachment or judgment allows us to develop an internal curiosity. As observers, we become neutral to the object of our observation. It's our awareness that makes this possible and illuminates the way. As we shine light upon the questionable areas within us with consciousness and curiosity, each step on the path gradually reveals itself like dense clouds dissipating to disclose a sun that has never stopped shining.

What, then, might we find as the path clears? What might we enlighten within us as we disentangle our identities from our emotions? In how many ways can we free our hearts? How much more does our project change when we recognize that we're neither our emotions nor our deepest wound? Rather, these are their own entities, aching to express themselves and be seen through the light of awareness.

Through their myth and folklore, many of the world's ancient civilizations described this life of ours as a great unfolding drama. The same can be said of our internal world, the microcosm within us. Yogic work teaches us to develop a different relationship with our consciousness. It encourages us to see our awareness as a bright light that projects the unexplored, unfolding drama of our deep emotions and habitual patterns onto the screen of consciousness. It invites us to take front-row seats and learn from what we see play out, in the guest house of our being.

By simply observing the emotion, we acknowledge its presence. By naming it (saying, *Oh, this is sadness. Hello, sadness*), we identify it as separate and extrinsic from our identity. Becoming a witness for our internal experiences provides a stage, a voice, and an audience for what has been silenced within us. In so doing, we create freedom for what was previously censored. In liberating our hidden emotional spaces through recognition and naming, we release ourselves from those very emotions and the ensuing habits they perpetuate. This is the beginning of waking up. The next step is to provide a safe and controlled space for the drama within us to tell its story. This is the art and craft of allowing.

13

THE POWER OF LETTING BE

SHIFTING FROM RESISTANCE TO ALLOWING

There are times in our lives when events feel balanced: when there's a flow to our work and our relationships; when we are filled with ease, joy, and the sense of *there's nowhere else I'd rather be at this moment*. This is our natural state, born out of experiencing the connection more than the disconnection, and the result of seeing more truth than untruth. Then there are times when everything is a struggle; when a move in any direction feels trying, all options seem hopeless, and even getting up in the morning feels like going against the grain of life itself. Although the former are moments of truth, it's within the state of struggle that the potential for our deepest learning is most present. These are the moments that call for our allowing.

Some of our most ingrained, conditioned patterns are clinging and grasping. Both are a form of attempted control. Times of non-flow in our lives are most often characterized by clinging—to a sensation, emotion, person, job, living situation, or ideal. These times are also characterized by grasping for that which we don't have; when we believe the possession of what we lack would create a higher level of happiness in our lives. We have built structures in our minds of how things "should" go—what our lives, partners, children, jobs, and schedules "should look like"— and it's clinging to those structures that keeps the wheel of our patterned suffering spinning. "Shoulds" exist only in one place—the mind. Again, the familiar motif emerges: We suffer when what we want or expect things to be like is other than what is in front of us at this moment. When we cling to how things "should" be, we stop them from opening themselves up; we fail to see, and hence learn from, the truth of their *actual* existence.

Philosopher Martin Heidegger said that truth is not a static object, a noun, but rather it is a happening, a verb. Heidegger presents truth as a dynamic unfolding toward authenticity and self-disclosure. For authenticity to develop, however, it necessitates what he called "a field of openness." In other words, the truth of who we are is not a fixed essence, but an open space of non-judgment, without others' or our own expectations.

Say, for example, all you want to do when you grow up is to be involved in the arts, but your parents are set on you being an engineer because it's the family trade. It's very likely that if you aren't true to your passion for art and don't find an outlet for its expression, you'll live as though there's something unfulfilled within you—a constant ache for something more. Isn't this urging common to our experience? Such a yearning might continue to call to us until it becomes urgent enough to disappoint the "shoulds" our parents have preemptively set out for us, and we decide to take a risk and explore our authentic interest. Otherwise, we may live with that deep denial for our own expression.

How different would our experience be if the people in our lives supported the development of our expanding authenticity and encouraged us to explore the areas within us that are filled with curiosity, without instilling a preconceived idea of what we should be, how we should act, or what should make us happy?

Because yoga is ultimately about removing the layers that don't allow us to see clearly, it's very much about removing the "shoulds," and in their place laying out a field of openness that promotes exploration and growth in ourselves, in others, and in life situations. In this space of open acceptance, we see these three elements for what they are, rather than as defined by the shackles that we've created and cling to—the chains of "shoulds" that keep us captive to inauthenticity.

Truth, allowing, and surrender go hand in hand, just as clinging, grasping, untruth, resistance, and suffering are all in the same camp. We already know that in times of flow we are our most authentic selves. In this space, we allow for experiences to transpire without holding on, and we allow people to be themselves without taking it personally. We aren't threatened by their journey. In flow, union, yoga, and joy, letting go comes easy because we're standing in what matters: the unchanging truth of who we are.

Alan Watts likens human experience to being immersed in an ocean. The waves thrash us around, when we happen to notice a large rock also tossed around by the waves. We have two options: hold on to the rock or not. Holding on to what might appear like a steady object that will support us during the turmoil may initially seem like a good idea, but ultimately the rock will sink to the bottom of the ocean and take us along with it. Watts suggests that in order to survive—to thrive—we must instead learn to float. We must learn to ride the waves and surrender our false sense of security.

In clinging to our structures and resisting what is before us, we become rigid. In flow, we are present to each wave as it comes, and instead of creating a dam that will eventually break with the pressure, we allow the waves to be as they are. In so doing, their very movement teaches us to surf. Likewise, every decision we have before us either supports allowing or clinging; it either bolsters the most authentic version of others and ourselves or negates it through resistance—fighting for people and circumstances to conform to a predetermined picture we've created in our minds.

Every action, word, and thought we put into the world either supports authenticity and promotes peace or supports falsehood and promotes pain. The degree to which we choose authenticity—allow ourselves, people, and experiences in our lives to unfold as they may; that is, the degree to which we surrender our resistance to life's unfolding—is directly proportional to the degree of peace and joy we will experience in our lives at any given moment. To understand and embody this truth is the key to our freedom and to lasting happiness. It is, no doubt, a task that requires substantial training. It requires us to learn the capacity to allow and develop the strength to fully surrender.

Allowing is the craft we develop, just as an illustrator might sketch various subjects over and over to gain insight on where she needs to improve her skills and sharpen them through repeated practice. Surrender is the finished masterpiece, the result of all the work, the epicenter of allowing. There are three main places where we can observe our resistance and practice our craft of allowing: ourselves, others, and life circumstances that are out of our control. As we do the work, change transpires, and ultimately the sweet relief of surrender becomes available.

14

ALLOWING THE SELF

THE CURSE OF THE SECOND ARROW

Allowing emotions to be expressed can be particularly difficult. Most of us find allowing downright uncomfortable. It requires endurance, and like any other skill, we need to develop expertise through practice and mistakes. Ironically, the task in itself is straightforward: Can you sit with the named, identified emotion and simply let it be, watch it, and allow it to unfold without taking action? When an emotion arises and you have identified it, can you watch the multitude of reactive tendencies that arise? These might be verbal or physical responses, or images in the mind of fleeing or retaliation. Can you bear witness to the truth of these emotions without reacting?

In shifting our role from experiencer to observer of the emotion, we've effectively altered how we relate to that emotion, and perhaps even how we relate to the event (or series of events) that led to it. Whereas we may have a reaction to an event, we also, primarily, have a relationship to that reaction. Say, for instance, that someone broke the side window to our car and stole the radio. For the sake of simplicity, let's also say that the main emotion that arises is intense anger. Our immediate reaction might be a desire to physically lash out, or to yell violent curse words. In that moment, we're in the center of the emotion where there is no space: we are in the belly of the beast, engulfed by reactive feelings. The anger could, if we let it, entangle us deeper and maybe compel us to take matters into our own hands and retaliate in some way.

Alternatively, we could notice the way in which we are relating to the anger. In the noticing, space immediately appears. Moreover, we can name the emotion (*Wow, I am very angry right now*) and let ourselves sit and explore the physicality of that emotion. We can allow ourselves to notice the heartbeat and breath speeding up. In that pause, the relationship to the anger changes. We have positioned ourselves in a completely different vantage point.

It might be helpful here to recall one of the primary insights of yogic wisdom: because things and events as they are bear the meaning we ascribe to them, our experience is mostly comprised of the quality of our relation to events rather than of the events themselves. Being entrenched in anger is qualitatively much different than being able to state how we feel and allowing that experience to be, and eventually, to pass. Hence the triggering event itself will be intrinsically and qualitatively changed. Our experience of life is altered, even if the event remains the same.

We can also bear in mind that the instantaneous emotional response is often a trigger to a larger wound that still hurts. If, for example, I owned a nice car, a symbol of my status, I might react differently to the break-in than someone whose automobile is vandalized and thinks, *I'm so lucky I wasn't here when this happened; I could have gotten hurt.* The person for whom the car symbolized an aspect of their self-concept (i.e., *I am successful, and this car represents my success*) is likely to experience more anger, frustration, and negative emotions at the crime because the crime will feel like a personal attack. Someone for whom the car is merely a means of transportation and not connected to his or her identity might not take the robbery so personally, and the quality of the emotional response will be less intense and negative.

Examining our reactions and learning to provide space for our emotions enlightens us about our level of attachment, possibly to people or situations we may not have realized we were identifying ourselves with. Learning to allow is a path to healing because it changes how we relate to an event that arouses intense emotion—and changes how we relate to our emotions themselves. Allowing is in effect a de-escalator of our triggers because it creates a necessary pause between event and reaction; in this space, consciousness arises. The space of allowing provides us an opportunity to reconnect with the present truth: We are here, now, tethered to this moment. Furthermore, allowing an emotion to exist without reaction helps us detangle events and attachments from our concept of self. With enough practice, we can learn to reconstruct our relationships with the events, people, and memories that ail us so that they no longer hold the powerful emotive control over us that tends to propel us backward into past pains or forward into future fears. We are effectively learning to redefine ourselves, emancipated from our triggers.

As we hone the craft of allowing, we're training our minds to become watchful when an uncomfortable or intense experience arises. The more we practice sitting with emotion, the less we get caught in its momentary flurry, and the more we learn the truth of its transience: Emotions and intensity *will* pass, and the more we simply allow them to be, the more easeful their passing becomes. In effect, we're training ourselves to shift from reactivity (a space of non-choice and identification with that which isn't actually us) to observance (a place of choice and freedom).

There may be some initial challenges to our work of allowing. We may find resistance to it in the first place, which, ironically, is most effectively explored through further observation. Resistance often shows up as that voice inside that says, *Nah, you don't need to meditate*. It's that list of excuses that keeps us from a task we know will benefit us. Yet, exploring resistance can be as simple as having a conversation with the resistance. When the voice says, *I don't have time to meditate*, you might reply, *Well, what if I make time?* It might respond, *You are simply just too busy*, to which you might say, *Well, if I can spend twenty minutes on social media, I can spend ten minutes sitting in stillness*. Or you can reply, *Well, what bad thing will happen if I meditate for ten minutes and run out of time later?*

As an experiment, you might see where the conversation goes, inquiring as to the elements of the resistance, and see if you can pare down the underlying feeling, perhaps to a word or phrase. (We will touch on more specific exercises in the Workbook.) Oftentimes, we find that underlying the resistance is self-judgment that may be keeping us from sitting with ourselves.

The Buddha once said that in life we cannot always control the first arrow. However, the second arrow is optional. The original pain over which we have no control is the first arrow, fired at us by life circumstances. Our first reaction to pain or discomfort isn't the underlying issue: so long as we are human, we are likely to react. Instead, the issue is the relationship to that emotion, or what happens next. In other words, we have the tendency to deny or cover up those emotions, or simply pile on a second layer—guilt for our grief, anger for our sadness, or the sensation of *I shouldn't be feeling like this*. This is the second arrow, and it's optional. How we respond to the second arrow is where allowing has the potential to transform itself into surrender: unadulterated release of the need to judge what we feel. We surrender our sense of "should" toward our own experience, and just like emotion, when we let it be, it softens and the intensity decreases.

Frequently, the second, third, and fourth arrows come so quickly that we may not even notice they're there. In the process of allowing our emotions to be as they are without reacting to them, we may find we have deeply held judgments about ourselves and the way we feel. We make grand generalizations: *Why am I so emotional? Why does everything make me so angry?* or *I wish I didn't want to punch a wall.* We can't fully witness, address, or allow the original emotion to pass when it's being shielded by a thick layer of judgment. We cannot appear to ourselves as we truly are, nor can we heal the wound left by the first arrow, when we're constantly shooting ourselves with subsequent arrows. Unless we learn to create a field of openness for ourselves without the confines of preconceived "shoulds," the second and third arrows, etc., will continue to pierce us.

The second arrow also stops us from connecting with ourselves, with others, and with our environment by keeping us from the moment at hand. Say, for example, that you broke your diet and ate a brownie during lunch. The self-blame of *Why did I do that?* or *Why wasn't I strong enough to resist the temptation?* replays in your mind while your body is trying to have a conversation with a friend, focus on work, or enjoy a piece of music. We can't access the underlying cause (i.e., the addiction to sugar) when we're spending our time in the blame game of the reaction because there's no problem that can be solved while we are still entrenched within the energy of said problem. All healing, by its very nature, requires space.

Once we awaken to the harms of the second arrow and to our predisposition toward shooting ourselves, we can take care of our self-inflicted wounds. With time, we learn how not to shoot that second arrow of self-criticism at all, and instead observe and tend to the underlying cause of pain. Through the practice of continual observing and allowing, we recognize that it's best to meet ourselves and our experiences not with weapons drawn, but on our knees with open arms.

15

ALLOWING AND RELATIONSHIPS

WALKING EACH OTHER HOME

A symbiotic relationship exists between our ability to allow within ourselves and our ability to hold that same space for others. As we develop one, the other is also enlarged; as we struggle in one, the other is affected. Yet, some find the internal work within the self more abstract, and the work in relationships more tangible. Relationships—whether casual, intimate, familial, or platonic—are intrinsic to our human experience. We're inherently relational beings, and unless we are pure ascetics, it's likely our lives are embedded in a matrix of relationships that inform our well-being. The craft of allowing and the art of surrender are especially relevant in how we relate to one another, and reciprocal to the amount of freedom or restriction we feel in our relationships.

Although relationships can be one of the most joyous aspects of being alive, they also can be filled with frustration, disappointment, betrayal, and other forms of suffering. Relationships are mediated through the yin/yang, coming/going, giving/receiving that happens between parties; the more intimate the relationship, the more important this balance becomes. When the scale is tipped for too long to one side, one person may feel hurt, unseen, unheard, or unfulfilled. When one party behaves in a way that the other experiences as wrong, the hurt party suffers and the tendency to control (the opposite of allowing) arises.

The yogic teachings suggest that the desire to control turns on like a lightbulb when things aren't as we want them to be. Let's recall that suffering occurs when we want something other than what is presently here, and control is a learned mechanism to cope with the suffering that emerges from this mental state. When a person behaves or reacts in a way we find off-putting, our internal alarm for self-preservation goes off.

Although we may think we're reacting to a person's behavior, we are in fact reacting to our internal alarm that announces: *Things are not how I want them to be right now!* As a result, we may find ourselves with racing hearts and frazzled thoughts, giving ultimatums, creating restrictions for the other person, saying or doing hurtful things in retaliation, or even shutting down to the other entirely.

This range of responses is reactivity, and it tends to make matters worse. Inherent in reactivity are anxiety and fear. Our nervous system is sending warning signals to the brain, and the intensity of our experience is heightened: it feels as though the problem we're facing is larger than life. Thus, we react from a place of self-preservation (based on the premise that we are not okay) and our behavior tends to be destructive to both the health of the relationship and ourselves.[18]

It's important to recall another of the basic yogic principles that applies here: So long as we are living from a place of *I am not okay*, we are caught in pain and its story. Yet, in truth, so long as we're not in actual danger, we *are* okay in this moment (even if we haven't been in the past). Locating where our feelings of not being okay operate from and recognizing they are caught in the web our mind is busy spinning are essential to the realization that reactivity is our mind replaying a story of the past.

Just as a dog who might get instantly excitable at the sound of a doorbell can be trained that there's no impending threat and to sit quietly and wait for the guest to enter the home, our responsive alarm can also be soothed and turned into watchfulness rather than instantaneous attack. (The Workbook will delve deeper into specific exercises designed to train reactivity.)

The second response is the seed of our conditioning. Reactivity and control (wanting to change what's happening or change another person) really stem from a fear of separation. Let's recall that the meaning of yoga itself is the ever-present yoking of experience, the realization of a constitutional unity that exists at all times in all beings: everything is always united. Always. No exceptions. When we find ourselves in a situation where someone behaves in a way that causes us to feel hurt, this is experienced as separation. We may no longer feel like we matter to this person: isolated, unheard, unappreciated, or unvalued. Suffering emerges as a result (whether it manifests as sadness, anger, frustration, etc. depends on each individual). Although it's the greatest fear we have, separation is the strongest illusion we subscribe to, cloaking the truth of our innate unity. If our suffering is based on the actions of another person, then it necessarily means that we aren't seeing something clearly, that our vision is tainted.

As an example, let's say that someone has lied to us about something important. We find out the truth and feel misled and betrayed. The pain here stems from the feeling of separation that the action of lying has stirred in us. We hold certain expectations in our relationships, and honesty and trust are fundamental building blocks of any healthy relationship. When, through lying, another person paints a picture that is different from the way things factually are, we base our actions on that false world. Finding out the truth can be extremely confusing: We are melding two realities, redefining words and actions in a brand-new context, and reinterpreting our reality.

In the process, we feel isolated. The isolation occurs for the period of time spent recontextualizing and letting our mental space catch up to the actuality of the situation. Whereas it's important to gain a clear picture so we can then behave accordingly, it's not like us to simply stop there. Instead, our (perhaps justifiable) tendency is to revisit the issue to try to "figure out" what happened, and whether it's likely to happen again.

It's common for victims of lies or betrayal to repeatedly ask the same questions, rerun the situation in their minds, and explore all avenues to ensure the truth. This is the space where we can get easily caught and where we perpetuate our pain. For as long as we fiddle with a reality in our mind, we miss the reality unfolding in front of us. In extreme cases of traumatic experiences that result in, say, symptoms such as flashbacks, the victim actually loses track of present reality and is momentarily convinced that the threat of the past is in the present. Unhealed, this gap between the mental experience and the ever-transpiring reality in front of us continues to expand and the suffering deepens. The same is true for less acute examples, such as lying. The result is that although the judgment and behavior of the party who lied affected us initially, the pain is perpetrated by our state of perceived isolation. The perpetuation and degree of the pain further depend on our capacity to return to the center of our experience in the present moment: to connect with what's here, in the home of our hearts.[19]

The fact that the perpetuation of our pain lies primarily in our hands doesn't minimize other people's abilities to be hurtful. Nor does it mean that people aren't responsible for their words and actions—they absolutely are. In fact, taking responsibility for our own behavior is part of the healing process. Instead, we need to recognize that, first, the behavior that causes pain stems from pain, meaning that if someone is acting in a legitimately harmful way, that behavior is stemming from their own sense of separation. No one (psychotic illnesses aside) who abides in a space of inner joy has the need to hurt others. Even inadvertent pain tends to arise out of internal conflict. Secondly, the way out of our pain lies in our ability to shift focus from the blame we place on others back to the seed of our own experience. Instead of blaming and resisting each other, we can train ourselves to observe and allow. This is where the magic—the learning, the healing, and ultimately the loving—happens.

There is one more element to consider in the conversation on betrayal and being hurt by another. Each of us is walking down a unique road, one made up of elements particular to our experience. Yogic philosophy suggests that this road is the path to, and the development of, our own authenticity—the truth of who we are. In walking this road, we're all experimenting with varying levels of authenticity: exploring what feels good and what doesn't, what frees us and what holds us down. The *Sūtras* say that all suffering is a result of ignorance, and the definition of ignorance is mistaking the painful as pleasant, the unreal as real, and (most centrally) the non-self as self—meaning that all ignorance essentially stems from not knowing ourselves.[20]

Hence, the road to self-knowledge is often potholed with ignorant pursuits—relationships, activities, and identities that feel good at first but which later (months, years, decades) we realize are terrible for us: diversions from our attempt to find home. In the end, we might not have had this insight if we'd not waylaid ourselves with ignorance. In retrospect, we can look back at a younger version of ourselves (hopefully with some lightheartedness) and say, *Oh, goodness. What was I thinking?* As we mature in our self-knowledge, the need to dive headfirst into the sea of ignorance decreases. Eventually, we just need to wade in knee-deep, then only dip a toe in. One day, all we might wish to do is look at the water and say, *No, that doesn't serve me.*

Through the course of our journey, we're inevitably bound to irritate some people (we are, after all, merely human!). Our actions necessarily create ripples in the lives of others. This is what Heidegger liked to call the "facticity" of others' existence. Our words and behaviors create facts that others must negotiate as they walk down their own path. To change the metaphor, our words and actions are like paintbrushes and paint that we use to create the world around us, a world that others are also a part of. It's guaranteed that we'll paint an inaccurate picture for another person, and hence create pain for them, whether we intend to or not. So how does this relate to allowing?

The principle of allowing in relation to the Other is at its essence a recognition that the path of another is as important as our own, and that we will inadvertently and inevitably step on each other's toes. Yet, our goal is to create space for it so that we may, as the *Sūtras* say, accept the unavoidable pain of this journey as growth without continuing its cycle.[21] As such, the principle of allowing as it pertains to the Other requires us to recognize that others' paths are a road toward their own authenticity, and that they're as fallible as we are. This is the foundation of compassion.

No area is perhaps more equipped to help us develop allowing than our relationships, for it's there that our efforts to control are most exasperated and our reactivity is most sensitive. Hence, our relationships can teach us the most about compassion. The tendency to control or coerce creates barriers for both parties in a relationship. It creates barriers for us as the controller because we wish to mold another person to fit our expectations, and for others because it limits their inherent freedom. If we took the seat of the witness with a curious heart that didn't look to take the actions of others as defining our own experience—if we didn't catastrophize another's words or behaviors but saw them instead as steps that person was taking toward their personal authenticity—then instead of jumping into our habitual reactivity, we'd acknowledge that we all carry within us unmet needs and that in order to fulfill them we need to be heard, seen, and accepted. What insights and freedom might both parties experience when we look at one another with curiosity and compassion and honestly consider, *In what way is _____ not being heard or seen? In what way can I witness their growth?*

The challenge, as always, is to observe the unfolding of ourselves and of the Other in nonjudgmental space. Oftentimes, this is enough to allow the observer effect to occur, and the Other feels our grip loosen. This loosening might not happen the first, second, or third time, but eventually it will become clear to the Other that our intent is no longer to control, but rather to connect from a space of mutual authenticity.

Here, the space between us and the Other is like a garden in which the buds of our most genuine selves can blossom, and true compassion for another's experience—for *their* suffering and pain—can grow. Eventually, allowing will become our primary mode of operation—wanting to connect with the Other's truths—and the chains of desire to control loosen.

If our relationships are to be based on truth and love, then what better approach is there than the gift of our presence to aid in another's growth? When we offer to help another's spirit open to authenticity, it's as if we're watching a flower bloom without forcing its petals into a shape they aren't ready to take. If we approach another as a still-unfolding flower, then what might our own efflorescence look like when we learn to appreciate others exactly where and how they are at the present moment? And what might happen within us when we can extend the same grace to ourselves? Imagine feeling not coerced but carried through our interactions; heard and seen through the act of supporting, hearing, and seeing the Other? What if part of this experience of living is learning to grow one another through our collective experiences, to bear witness to each other's shedding of the layers of inauthenticity and false seeing so we can then become like clean mirrors for each other's light and guides for each other's awakening? I believe this is what Ram Dass meant when he said, "We are all just walking each other home."

16
EQUANIMITY
ALLOWING LIFE TO UNFOLD

The principle of allowing is also applicable to events in our lives. In the face of circumstances beyond our control, we tend either to hold on tighter or project our need to control onto other arenas. Life contains countless uncertain circumstances: career changes, geographic relocations, health issues, and divorces, among many more. Although we can do a lot in each one of these arenas, it can feel as though our fate lies in the hands of forces greater than our own. Most of us have experienced having to wait for a life-altering decision to be made by a third party, over whom we have no control. Many of us have faced shocking news that instantly changed the course of our lives. When we take a moment to consider the breadth of experiences possible, we should be humbled by the transpiring coincidences that have brought us to where we are today, and the sheer magnitude of how much isn't in our control. This humility can carry with it existential angst, and may overwhelm us.

As we've explored, yogic wisdom teaches us that the crux of any situation is not in the situation itself, but in how we relate to it. Freedom or captivity in any circumstance depends on how tightly we're bound to the discomfort that arises in the face of instability, how locked in we feel to the potential outcomes. It's not that we're expected to not have *any* reactions. If we find out we're being laid off or that a loved one is critically ill, we'll naturally react, and the immediate period after the reaction might be filled with many different emotions as we grieve our losses. Yogic wisdom isn't suggesting that things should be any different. Instead, it teaches us how to regain equilibrium. This is often referred to as equanimity.

Equanimity consists of learning to return to truth, to ourselves, and to a place where we can connect with our wholeness. True to the pattern of our human conditioning, equanimity can be learned through self-knowledge and practice. The truth, yoga teaches, is that the entire natural world is based in movement, a dance always in motion. Our clinging for stability speaks to the places within us that feel unstable. Some of us are more shaken by instability in our living situations, others by instability in our careers or relationships. These are keys to greater self-knowledge, and greater self-knowledge decreases our ignorance and hence our sensation of disconnectedness.

The work of equanimity can happen by reflecting on times in our lives when we felt hopeless, least in control, and unable to get back up. Through reflection, we can learn where our wounding lies. The work toward healing these wounds continues to be the same: We come back to the present moment, take on the witnessing seat, pay close attention to our reactions, name them, and allow them to breathe in a space of non-judgment and non-action.

In the face of instability or sudden change, we can observe our reactions to different types of instabilities and notice the following: Which have a tighter hold on our sense of freedom? Which ones leave us feeling like we have no options, chained to the circumstance at hand? Can we adopt the seat of the witness and create the stage of allowing upon which we simply observe the circumstances of our life develop? Can we give those circumstances the very freedom that we long for? When all that we can do has been said and done, can we cultivate a time to listen and observe, and from there allow the next step to manifest effortlessly?

If, you may ask, we feel as if we have no choice in a developing circumstance in our lives, then how can we say "don't do anything," if we can't do anything anyway? The "doing" to which I'm referring is both physical and mental. The principle of witnessing and allowing asks us to cultivate a space of stillness within which life can unfold. This isn't to say that we ignore the situation; in fact, quite the opposite: We must pay special attention to what is happening within us (our emotions, bodily sensations, fears, and hopes for the future based on the situation, our memories of the past that the situation arises) and watch. We become mindful of what we say about the topic, and recognize and cease the projections (particularly negative ones) of what might happen. Instead, we let the circumstance unfold in the moment and allow decisions to be made at the time they are required. In the meantime, we rest with what transpires without jumping to conclusions.

Over time, the stillness of observation expands our capacity to allow and lessens the stress during the waiting period, and we become better acquainted with the quality of equanimity. We learn, too, that equanimity feels freeing. When we turn our attention away from our expectations or potential catastrophic outcomes and instead toward our experience with compassion and openness, our perspective changes. When we feel space within ourselves, the expectations for the situation loosen, and we regain our composure. When we're composed, we're able to return to what exists at the present moment, freed from the captivity of future-thinking and anticipating.

There's a simple test to detect equanimity: We can observe how our physiological state (breathing patterns, heart rate, etc.) differs when we anticipate catastrophic outcomes versus when we have a stable, present mind. The qualitative difference between these experiences is priceless. At the heart of equanimity lies the treasure of surrender. We can only bounce back to the present when we release expectation and attachment to the outcome of any situation. We can only get back up when we let go of the ground.

Through witnessing and allowing, we transform control into compassion, aversion into support, and pain into yet another step toward the revelation of our truest, unchanging nature. The more we create space within us, the more it happens effortlessly. We take the actions of others less personally, we interpret life as happening *to* us less, and we perceive people to be hurting us less. We experience life as it is—a beautiful experiment in authenticity, a challenging and rewarding game we get to play together, where we're all walking the road to opening our hearts, to being as we truly are. To succeed in the game, we must master the most challenging of skills and defeat the most vicious of opponents: forgiveness and fear.

17
SURRENDERING AND FORGIVENESS
THE SHIFT FROM FEAR TO LOVE

Surrender and the Physical Body

I'm admittedly an *āsana* junkie; I think many "yoga people" are. It's no mystery to me why, of all the different elements and types of yoga (*bhakti*—the yoga of devotion; *karma*—the yoga of selfless action; *jñāna*—yoga through studying texts and wisdom in order to distinguish the self from the non-self; *japa*—the yoga of repetition of names and mantra), it is *haṭha* and more specifically *āsana*, the yoga of postures, that has exploded in the West. In my home of Manhattan, yoga studios are popping up like flowers rising out of the earth during an especially fruitful spring season. On the internet, I see advertisements for yoga teacher trainings almost daily: FULFILL YOUR DREAM. BECOME A YOGA TEACHER. As soon as the practice of postures went viral, its profit-making potential was revealed and *voilà*: everyone and their cousins are now yoga teachers.

Back in the days of my first training, you'd be hard-pressed to find a teacher who took you in without three to five years of practice under your belt. It was common to undergo a lengthy interview process before being accepted to a training program. At the completion of a program, new teachers were required to teach at least a year for free: to give back what they'd been given, to cultivate the craft, and to practice the art of teaching. That was a liberal approach! Not too many years prior, teachings of yoga were considered esoteric, and teachers were veterans who'd practiced for decades with the great masters, and were utterly committed to this practice not as something they did for fitness or fun, but as a complete way of life.

Today, it's not uncommon for me to step into a yoga teacher–training to teach philosophy and encounter people who've only been practicing yoga for a few weeks before they decided to become a "teacher." The modern yoga landscape has changed drastically even in the last decade, and it will continue to transform as new teachers innovate new forms of yoga, and more and more people start their path in this practice of conscious movement.

I'm not pointing out the change in the yogic landscape to be dismissive. My aim is to bring light to an interesting dynamic: unlike the other forms of yoga—like the study of books, or feeding the poor, or chanting—*āsana*, postures and physical movement, stuck to Western culture and we can't seem to get enough. The Western mind is body-centered, our culture revolves around the acquisition of material goods, and our focus is on the feel and appeal of our physical bodies. Beauty, health, and success are often measured through physical standards. No wonder we've become *āsana* junkies!

Although wanting to look and feel good isn't necessarily negative (there's much to be said about the power of positive addiction), popular yoga culture may have lost sight of or perhaps never fully accessed the subtler layers of this amazing practice. The more I teach, and the more my own practice deepens, the more I'm convinced that we're not addicted to the postures themselves. We are addicted to the doors they open within us. *Āsana* has become a passage to the nuanced teachings of the practice, which is to say, to the deeper and richer places within ourselves, to the sensations of our aliveness that are generally imperceptible to the preoccupied mind and the stressed-out body. *Āsana* provides us with a very palpable, accessible, and corporeal experience of change and impermanence; it teaches us, from the very grounded space of our raw physicality, to surrender.

It is to these subtler places that much of this book is devoted. True to the *Sūtras*, my approach to the movement portion of the yogic practice is simple. The *Yoga Sūtras* dedicate only two threads to the physical practice of yoga, and they are straightforward: "Posture should be steady and comfortable," and "posture is mastered/attained by the release of effort and absorption into the infinite."[22] In other words, according to the sages, we find true posture when it is centered, easeful, and used as a tool to move beyond the body and into the infinite. This requires practice. Because of this, the practice of movement is relevant, and it's a helpful tool in teaching us about surrender. We cannot allow ourselves and our consciousness to be absorbed into the infinite if we're still mulling over our grocery list in triangle pose, or holding on to a resentment in our walking-around-daily pose—in our yoga *off* the mat.

Surrender, then, is necessary for yoga, but it's an elusive concept. When we ask the question, *How, exactly, do we let go?* there's no verbal answer, and no step-by-step procedure to follow. In fact, even when we imagine full surrender, it's evanescent: we grasp the notion for a second, but we're quickly pulled back into our circumstances. There is, however, one place where surrender is more tangible: in our physical bodies. Experiencing physical surrender then trickles down and within, like nectar into the vastness of our mind and the subtlety of our spirit.

In the practice of *āsana*, surrender is most exemplified by the last, and perhaps most important, posture of all: *savāsana* (dead man's pose/final relaxation). After an hour or two of labor, of digging and pushing, of aligning and moving, of staying with the rhythm of our breath, of guiding the mind away from problems, aches, and pains, *savāsana* allows us to surrender completely. It doesn't happen every time, or even half of the time, but it's magical when it does. Surrender is the complete dissolution of previous misgivings, belief systems, heartaches, and even muscular tightness. It's the expression of absolutely yielding to what's here now. It's the respite that arrives after the final brick of our internal walls has been removed. Surrender is healing. It's also a choice, and we may need guidance getting there.

It's my belief that to a large degree, the rise in popularity of yoga and yoga teacher–trainings stems from a place within us that wants others to know the depth of surrender we've gotten to touch because of our practice. It's like we're Lucy and we've discovered the magic wardrobe into Narnia in *The Lion, the Witch, and the Wardrobe*, and we want to take others there, so that they, too, may experience the possibilities. (This gives me hope for our future as a civilization!) In the face of a harsh world, it is as noble as it is necessary that we help one another wake up and let go—and every little bit helps. What if we lived in a world where we were all working to tear down the walls that limit our self-concepts, that make us reactive and closed off, and we spent more time simply surrendering? This is perhaps the most fundamental question that the earnest teacher (and student) of yoga asks themselves.

Nonetheless, I don't believe that the practice of *āsana* is uniquely different from other practices in its ability to bring us to our breaking point, or to place us in front of our own existential mirror. Nor is it the only practice that enables us to achieve that full and exhaustive experience of complete and utter surrender. I've personally found surrender in the most unlikely places—martial arts, writing, and parenting all require the sweetest and hardest of surrenders. And in all these practices, it's when you surrender that you strike gold.

What these activities have in common in my personal life is that I'm a practitioner of all three. I show up on a regular basis and spend time in study and devotion with the practice. I (figuratively) slam my head against a wall when the practice frustrates me to no end. I push myself to show up when I can make up every excuse in the world not to. I've spent enough time in the commitment to each of these practices that I've dug myself into a hole of self-doubt, and in those times the practice has met me and become a ladder out.

Practice—whether it's of *āsana*, martial arts, painting, running, a relationship, or parenthood—is a commitment that requires complete presence and wholeheartedly asks us to look within. Then, it makes the biggest request of all: It asks us to let go. We can surrender from exhaustion, heartache, disappointment, and feeling absolutely beat-up, and from the failure of our expectations staring us in the face. Surrender can be like falling down a well. Then, you simply stop. You land. You are still. In the fall, the expectations, doubts, and debasements have also fallen. It's then that we release into the sweetest of faiths—the act of surrendering it all despite every reason not to. Despite life itself.

What makes yoga unique, however, is that in this practice we explicitly address and study surrender. We deliberately come to its door, knocking. Patañjali wasn't shy about it: the very first *sūtra* of his second book, which relates entirely to how we turn philosophy into practical application, says that yoga in practice consists of three elements: self-discipline, study, and surrender.[23] What makes yoga unique is that each practice is a training in surrender, to see just how much we can let go—and pay attention to the result.

For instance, we may find that in taking *savāsana* we tend to see more of why we *don't* allow ourselves to let go. The practice has somehow made the voices, the internal chatter, and the continual lists in our heads louder. We lie on our mats or on our meditation seats and everything that shouldn't be turned up, is. So, in that session we may not have "surrendered," but we've learned what surrender is *not*. We learn what is keeping us tied to drama, what dramas we are replaying, and which have a special hold on us. And that is a lot to learn in one day. We are honing our *viveka*, our discernment.

Surrender has always reminded me of an invisible ghost that leaves me wondering if it's a folktale or real. But I assure you, surrender is real; you just can't get to it through the brain, which is the way that I—and I think many of us—attempt to apprehend it. Like joy and love and other fundamentally human expressions that we endlessly deconstruct, surrender does not appear through force. Surrender comes when you surrender: a lovely tautology.

While we can't hurry surrender, we *can* make its arrival more welcoming. We can set the table and brew the tea; we can make our inner space warm and hospitable. We can clean up a bit, and it helps to take out the trash, because it stinks and it's near impossible to have a nice teatime with a pile of garbage nearby collecting flies. That pile of trash is fear. Although we may not know exactly when surrender will arrive, we do know that while fear is around, surrender won't be knocking on our door.

Fear: The Block and Key to Surrender

We don't let go because we're afraid. If we aren't letting go, by definition we are holding on, and if we are clinging on madly it's because we're afraid of what we can't control. Fear keeps us from surrender. Yogic practices help us get clear on what we're holding on to and maybe even why we've deceived ourselves into believing that we need whatever it is we can't let go of. It's improbable (or perhaps even impossible) for us to let go of something if we don't realize we're holding on to it in the first place, and so much of the time we are unaware, blind, and in denial of our own patterns, of our fear, guilt, and anger. But if we learn to see what's there, if we learn to discern the locks that keep us confined, we can more easily find the key to open them.

Everything we're afraid of is something we can't control—death, going broke, losing love—and every one of these things is a perceived separator. In death, we're separated from the living; in loss of financial security, we're separated from a life we're accustomed to; in losing love, well, that one is obvious and I think we all fear this one most. Fear is magnified isolation and its antidote is simple: remembrance.

This is what Marianne Williamson refers to as our "return to love." In the truth and unity of love there is no differentiation, and fear necessitates differentiation for its existence. Hence, in non-differentiation, where the ego is expanded so it merges with precisely what is in front of us at any given moment, there is no fear; there is only love. Letting go of fear is very much intertwined with letting go of our self-concepts, of unlearning so much of who we've come to believe ourselves to be, and paying attention to whatever it is that we're grasping at. When we do this, we shift from being a vulnerable and definitive entity to being a softer, wider, and less-defined entity. This is a state of being filled with more potential than actuality, like a seed ready to sprout, unattached and unafraid.

Letting go of fear doesn't mean not having fear. Instead, it means letting trust abide within us *despite* the sensation of fear. Eventually, the light of trust and surrender outshines the darkness of fear. Fear has a number of qualities and ways in which it manifests. It can reside within us in a way that hardens us and doesn't let anything else in, or it can affect our behavior through controlling others or our circumstances (e.g., *I was hurt by love and promise to never fall in love again, so I will no longer date*). But fear can also be the key to hope, perhaps especially when it's at its darkest.

In fact, fear can be so overwhelming and all-consuming, and can create such an unbelievable mess of us, that it becomes the conduit *to* love, to asking for help, and to surrendering. Anne Lamott says that it's when we cry out in our deepest desperation, when we are our most degraded and isolated, that we are also nice, tender, and teachable. In other words, our prayer tends to be the most sincere when we're on our knees begging for respite from the pain and the only words we can utter are "God, help me." This is the most powerful prayer of all. At some point, the fear becomes too much to bear and a miracle happens: we finally ask for help.

Asking for help is recognizing that we are, by nature, both limited and unlimited. We can't possibly see the whole picture, and yet we're intrinsically connected to a larger truth that can access the full spectrum and help us understand our place in it. Yogic philosophy suggests that our individuated consciousness (*prakṛti*) stems from and hence always has access to a non-differentiated field of consciousness (*puruṣa*). Our individual awareness is not separated from it; it is simply localized. Tapping into *puruṣa* is the religious/spiritual/creative experience. It's a means of realizing our egos are not the center, but a tiny jigsaw piece in a magnificent multi-dimensional puzzle. Pulling ourselves outside of the individualized ego for a moment can give us these glimpses of divine connection/synchronicity/creativity/realization. The prayer *God, help me*, or however we reach out to that which lies beyond ourselves, is a humble recognition of the limits of our understanding. It is okay to *not* know. It is even more okay to admit it. Prayer, then, is an invitation for our awareness to broaden, open, and tap into a glimpse of that magical picture of which we are both a minuscule and integral piece.

Prayer in this sense is an invitation not so much for the world or for our circumstances to be different than they are (it's not, *God, give me a million dollars!* or even,

God, please cure his cancer), but rather a plea for *us* to be different, for us to get a peek at a greater reality that will loosen the hold of our suffering, and will remind us of the incredible tenacity, vibrancy, and fullness of our souls, a reality that does not center on our limited understanding, but is a radical shift in perspective from the experience of our tiny selves into the greatness of the context that we are always, fundamentally and constitutionally, a part of. Prayer is asking for the wisdom to think, speak, and act in a way that's conducive to creating a peaceful space for all parties involved so we can zoom out of whatever misery or conundrum is presently consuming us, much like a spaceship taking off observes our magnificent planet shrinking until it's only a speck in the distance. In this distance is space; and in that space the grasp and intensity of suffering lessen. Prayer is asking for our perspective to be broadened like the space-ship's. It is requesting that our magnified and fixed sense of identity become more fluid and less resistant, so we can expand and connect—really, truly connect—with a more inclusive and more accurate vision of reality. Prayer is asking for our minds, and ourselves, to be greater.

The essence of prayer, then, is asking The Power (whose name is ultimately incon-sequential) to help us lift the veils (of *avidyā*—ignorance, non-seeing, wrong-seeing) that keep our perspective focused in on ourselves. Asking for help/prayer isn't about changing what is going on in our lives. The external world doesn't have to change for our situation to change—but our perspective does, and occasionally we need a little help with this task. Sometimes we just need to get hit over the head by a miraculous re-envisioning of things.

Shifting our perception from something we fear, hate, or resent into something we admire, have gratitude for, or eventually love, is nothing short of just that—a miracle—because through that shift we have been systematically altered. When it happens, our experience becomes so radically different that it can't help but have a greater effect all around, and our lives change. In other words, asking for our pettiness to go away is the same as asking for the suffering to cease. In the asking alone is a natural softening—when we ask for help we're vulnerable, ripe, defenseless, teary-eyed, and maybe even broken-down. But we have, in our beautiful, raw, snotty-nosed, messy, and imperfect way, arrived at the doorstep of surrender. We learn that fear can facilitate surrender, but it's not necessary to hit rock bottom every time. In fact, it's exhausting to do that. Some of us may need many occasions of falling on our faces in puddles of tears to come to this realization.

But it doesn't have to get so desperate, really, if we learn to work with fear and come to surrender more quickly—and, dare I say, more gracefully. As it turns out, there's a bit of a shortcut: learn to let go, despite (or because of) the fear. The fear can still be there, but let go of the attachment to it, and act as though it isn't there. Let go and ask for help to see that greater picture, with the awareness that encompasses more than just your tiny story. Let go and talk to the fear. Ask it what it's hiding, what it's trying to control, and then ask it to leave. Sometimes, it will talk back—so clearly, in fact, it's alarming and will give you goosebumps. It may have wise things to say about why we can't surrender. So, we can turn to fear and ask the fear itself to help and say, *Hey, what am I holding on to? What have I not forgiven? Show me, please.*

Forgiveness is a magical word. To forgive is to wipe the slate clean for others; but mainly, it's to wipe it clean for ourselves. Often, we're afraid because we haven't forgiven. Maybe we haven't forgiven our caregivers for doing what we felt was a lousy job at making us feel supported and loved, or our spouses for crossing a line they vowed they wouldn't, or our kids for being so damn ungrateful in the face of all our sacrifices. Sometimes, we don't realize what we haven't yet forgiven. Yet, when we explore and inquire within the deeper layers of ourselves and our work becomes subtler, we can get hit over the head with obvious realizations of what we haven't forgiven. We see what we haven't yet learned to accept, trust, or love. We comprehend that we're still viewing through the lens of our own shattered and wounded story, rather than through the magnificent openness that is available to us, if we only learn to soften and ask. Maybe we realize that it isn't someone else we're upset at, but rather that we haven't forgiven ourselves for giving up art, or dancing, or our dream of doing standup comedy.

The unforgiven ties us to the past, to things that are no longer actually real. Those ties keep us locked in the energy of the wound. When we have not yet forgiven, we carry with us the emotions of our past betrayals and use them as a building ground for our present relationships. When we bring the past into the present, we curtail the possibility for change and growth. If we are building new things with rusted tools and dilapidated materials, how reasonable is it to expect different results? If you take apart a house whose foundation was rotting, and use the same wood and nails to put it back together again, how can you expect a sturdy and habitable home? Forgiveness not only implies surrender, it necessitates it. It asks that we allow the past to remain in the past and the present to be reborn with all possibilities. Surrender implies forgiveness;

it imbues the present with the understanding that despite the past, the present gifts us new options. That, in fact, is the very offering that the present moment brings to us: a chance for rebirth.

Imagine if all trespasses, abuses, and betrayals you've experienced at the hands of others didn't alter the way you perceived other people or situations. Imagine if they were so insignificant that they were easily forgotten and easily forgiven. Even in considering that statement the ego may tighten, fight back, and say, *That was not unforgettable. That was painful!* No one is saying it wasn't painful; you're allowed that pain. But to not forgive is to build our lives over piles of pain.

Forgiveness is wiping our inner space clean by saying, *That wasn't the best version of you and so I will let it go, despite the suffering it might have created for me,* and (here's the hard part) meaning every single word of it. Forgiveness is identifying, *This pattern with this friend/partner/coworker seems to be cyclical. I forgive, but I choose to step away from this relationship.* Forgiveness doesn't require us to stay in the situation; it asks that we not carry it with us as we move forward; it asks us to begin anew.

In forgiving others, we're really gifting ourselves the space to heal and both the permission to feel hurt and to move on from that hurt. Unforgiveness is a labyrinth of bitterness within us that hides dead ends that can revert us back to our original hurt state. Walking out of the labyrinth is the equivalent of doing the very internal work we've been discussing—of becoming so familiar with that labyrinth that our continual acknowledgment and acceptance of it unwinds its path for us. It then becomes resoundingly clear that our unforgiveness and our bitterness—no matter how much it's directed at another person, no matter how justified it may feel—first and foremost abides within us. We are the primary seed of our emotions. The root and the home of what we give to others resides, at its genesis, always within us. And this is where it's strongest. Our primary job, then, is to tend to our own garden and fertilize our flowers with forgiveness so that they may bloom. When they do, we are released.

18
LOVE

I didn't feel it on the plane ride out west, but flying tends to distract me anyway. I find getting off the ground terrifying, and I used to require a hearty dose of downers before liftoff. I've learned to just breathe through that fear now, and it's painless, for the most part. Eventually, the rattling in the belly of the plane and that sinking feeling in the pit of my stomach stop and we've hit that altitude where you can see cities all at once over a broad, quilt-like terrain of grasses, asphalt, and fields you didn't know existed. Even if I expect such a vista, it surprises me every time: the way houses and buildings become little toys and grow smaller until they're only specks—miniature dots in a watercolor landscape, almost indistinguishable from one another, blurring into the background.

At about 25,000 feet I start to think about how tiny the buildings really are, about all the itty-bitty people that live and work in them, and how I know their worlds feel so large and important. They are, and yet they're not, all at once. I think about how our scale on the ground is so skewed most of the time and for so much of our lives.

Then the plane levels off and we're cruising at 40,000 feet. Now I can't see the buildings because we've zoomed out so far. All that exists is that amazing expanse of sky that's always there, but we forget just how magnificent it is, consumed instead with the gravity of our lives on the ground. Oh, but that sky is so much greater and so beautiful to look at, so freeing to be in! In this sublime vastness you get to take a break from and simultaneously catch a glimpse of how tethered to minutiae we are in relation to how much space exists. One senses how there's room for everything if we only managed to look up.

It feels wonderful to be among the clouds, so interesting to be alive to experience it, and for a moment grasp the actual magnitude of that very concept. Eventually, that feeling fades. It's almost funny (in that cosmically ironic sort of way) that in reality it's humanly impossible to live at this altitude; it's impractical to live zoomed out entirely, no matter how inspiring the view is. We must, to some degree, come down to earth, however much our human ingenuity has made it possible for us to touch those high places, if only momentarily.

I watch the clouds for most of the flight and observe how they gather from behind my small window, which is beginning to accumulate bits of frost along its rounded edges, forming a crystalline border around my breathtaking view. The clouds huddle like herds of sheep, then float on and disperse like bubbles at sea, evanescent as epiphanies—as if they'd never been there at all, as if someday they're sure to return.

When I first asked Mami where Papi had gone after he died, she pointed skyward. "He's in the clouds," she said, "with Johnny." I was eight years old and my favorite movie was a Johnny Appleseed cartoon Papi had gotten me for my birthday, where Johnny spent his days planting seeds, growing trees, and communicating with animals. At the end of the movie, Johnny dies, but we see his re-emergence in the sky, where he continues to plant trees in fields of clouds, little squirrels and antelope following close behind him. Mami told me that even if you move to heaven, the plants you sow on Earth keep growing. Whatever you planted takes root, she told me.

I remember flying to the United States as we left our native Colombia after Papi's death and looking for my father in the clouds, hoping he'd make an appearance or give me some sort of sign to let me know he was there, planting trees with Johnny. Even today when I fly, I still look out—for both of my parents this time—searching for a mild apparition, or a cloud resembling a fruit tree.

The fear began to creep in once I landed in San Francisco, and the feeling intensified as I signed the rental-car agreement, and continued to stir in the depth of my belly as I plugged the GPS into the port and typed in the address: 244 Concord Lane. By the time I hit the *d* my fingers shook gently. I took a deep breath. I had about three hours to compose myself, to relax into the experience I'd accepted—or more accurately, the experience I sought out. In Sanskrit, one of the words used to describe it is *tapaḥ*, that thing you know you must do. It might be excruciatingly uncomfortable, but it needs to get done if you're going to live with integrity.

It had been well over a decade since I'd seen or communicated with my guardians—since I'd stepped foot in that awful house, the one teeming with the distresses of my youth. It had also been about five years since my downfall and hospitalization, and since I'd found my practice, my yoga. In fact, it was my yoga that had instructed me to come back.

While my anxiety grew, I couldn't quite put my finger on what, exactly, I was afraid of. Was I worried that once I saw my guardians, the people I held responsible for so much of my suffering, I would just lose it? That despite my best efforts and hard work, I would scream and shout and throw things, the way they did at me more than ten years ago? Was I scared that they still held some power over me, still had the capacity to inflict punishment? Was I terrified that they were going to hurt me or lock me in a room with a man more than twice my age? Logically, I knew none of this would happen. Yet, there was an inkling of all these things somewhere in my emotions. Mainly, though, I just experienced an unnamed anxiety in my body.

I drove the three hours mostly in silence and entered the tiny Northern California town. I knew that town the way you know your most intimate friend, the way you can predict what they're going to laugh at or what they're going to say next. I drove its roads with the comfort of putting on an old pair of pajamas. I was here. I made the right turn onto Concord Lane, said a little prayer, and took a deep breath.

I knew that if I was going to complete my healing I had to face what I'd run away from for so long. I knew that I had done good work in those years of my healing, and I knew that if I was to talk or teach or write about the healing process, as I intended to do, I had to put my money where my mouth was, which in this case meant going back to Oakdale and seeing my guardians again. It meant coming face-to-face with my past, and with full presence actually forgiving my abusers.

Ron looked old and worn down, almost weak. "Hi there," I said. He greeted me and asked me to come in. "Would you like to see your old room?" he asked. I nodded. Stepping into the house was like stepping into one of those half-lucid dreams where you can watch a version of yourself doing something, but you can't control the scene. I saw my younger self in those rooms, the spotless floor, every knickknack cleaned to perfection. I looked down the hallway—a hallway that represented dread incarnate for me as a kid. I used to have nightmares about that hallway, about the way my guardians would walk down the long corridor, extending for what seemed like miles, looking for me, punishment imminent.

This was the hallway where I had my first panic attack at fourteen, the bathroom on the left where I was locked in without food, and where I first cut myself. On the far right was the room where the very man next to me pointed a gun at me, where I held my sister's passed-out body, and where I wished he would have just killed us both. It looked so . . . small. In fact, the whole house felt three times smaller than it did in my youth and in my memories. All of a sudden, the fear in my belly dissipated like the clouds outside the window of the plane.

Jenna wasn't there. It would be another five years until I'd face her again, until I found out that the whole time we lived in their home she knew that Ron was having an affair. She eventually left him after two decades of marriage. In that time, I would also come to find out that, as a child, Jenna was severely physically, emotionally, and sexually abused as well. It would be another several years until, in my position of domestic violence counselor, I realized there was a cycle of abuse between Ron and Jenna that I didn't have the insight to perceive while I was under their care. While advocating for victims of domestic violence, I also learned that abuse occurs in cycles, and those who have experienced it in childhood are statistically more likely to repeat it.

In the coming years I would also learn that Manuel had been deported and hospitalized in a mental institution back in Colombia after a psychotic breakdown. The man who stole my first encounter with sexuality was also a severely wounded person, now in shackles. It took all those years for me to gain a clear picture of the context of my childhood wounds pertaining to abuse, from a space that was other than the depths of my own isolated experience. Then, I came to the greatest realization of all: *It was never about me.*

In that meeting with Ron, on that summer day, there wasn't a long conversation about past sorrows, past betrayals, past bruises, or abuses. There wasn't screaming or yelling or throwing dishes; no knuckle sandwiches or big white fists around my jugular. There wasn't anything resembling my countless fantasies about punching my guardians in the face if I ever saw them again, or yelling, *How could you do the things you did?!* with my dukes in the air, demanding answers. There weren't any grand apologetic gestures or even a simple *I'm sorry* on his end. There was, in fact, no recognition of our shared and tattered histories. Instead, we engaged in small talk, as though a decade of silence had not just been broken. We sipped on lemonade as we chatted, and after a little while I said I had to be on my way. He got up to hug me. I hugged him back and said *goodbye*. That was the last time I ever saw Ron.

As a child, I remember watching Mami get dressed for work, the way a child admires everything a parent does. It always shocked me when she removed her shirt, the entirety of her back covered in thick scars, protruding lines and deep crevices running across her shoulders to the small of her back, like an ocean splintering into hundreds of tiny rivers that one day suddenly dried up.

When I grew a little older, I came to find out that when Mami was a little girl, her parents punished her by soaking her in a cold bath until her skin was soft and thin and then beat her with a horsewhip or with a wire hanger so that the pain would be more severe and so that the punishment would leave a mark, a reminder. Yet all I ever saw from Mami was love for her parents. In fact, she used to draw portraits of them, and when we lived in Colombia, she wrote them letters and recorded audiotapes for them constantly. *Mis viejitos*, she'd call them with tenderness, my little old ones.

I couldn't fathom how Mami was capable of so much soft love for the people who deformed her body in such a barbaric way, how she was capable of having such tender affection for the father who in a drunken fury kicked her so hard he split her shin. All over Mami's body were marks and scars with corresponding stories like these, like an old war zone with lingering remnants of the violence. One day I asked her, "How can you love them so much after what they did to you?"

Without skipping a beat, she said, "I forgave them."

"Did they ever apologize?" I asked.

"*Nunca*," she said. Not once.

I can't say with full honesty that I have the kind of love for my guardians that Mami did for her parents. But I can say that I've forgiven them, and that, in a sense, I have come to love that shattered past, the fear they once instilled in me, the sorrow that I went through as a result of abuse. Without it, I would never have realized the tenacity of my own heart, nor the resolve of the human spirit. And for that, I'm grateful. For that, I have deep love.

Love isn't only a spontaneous emotion that arises out of just the right circumstances, like staring into the eyes of our beloved over a candlelit dinner, or the natural effusion that springs out of us instinctively for a child, a sibling, or even our pets. It's true that love can flower effortlessly from these places. It's easy to love that which we cherish—a perfectly sunny day, kittens, the things and people that make us feel alive. But it's also true that we can teach ourselves to see and experience love in people and circumstances where it isn't so obvious, and where love feels quite difficult, even impossible to find. Places, people, situations that enrage or cripple us in fear are in fact the places where finding—read: *creating*—just a sliver of love makes all the difference.

It makes a miracle. It starts inwardly and it pours forth, expanding exponentially. Love isn't an isolated emotion: it's an attitude; a disposition; a *choice* that we can consciously make; a way of being that we can foster; and a muscle that we can strengthen through our behavior, our speech, and our thoughts. In fact, this is perhaps *the* ninja training of all the trainings—the *where can I create love in this situation* state of mind is the highest form of practice.

The work is reminiscent of Johnny Appleseed: training ourselves to see where we sow the seeds of love, what part of our garden we avoid, and what places need our tending the most. The work is identifying where we're resistant to planting and watering our love, and what barriers we have built, because of past pains, to keep us from that part of our garden, that part of ourselves. Then, the work involves going to those places, tearing down those walls, tilling the soil and planting the seeds anyway, watering them consistently, and plucking out the recurring weeds.

Or love is much like riding a bike. No matter how many books on riding we might read, we won't ever get any good at riding a bike until we climb on, start pedaling, and learn that delicate balance. Sowing and finding love is like anything else we might take on: we do it through practice. We practice to find the truth that if anything exists at all—no matter how rotten or disappointing or distressing—love exists within it simply because love is the essence of existence itself, of being-ness proper. In the spaces of resistance, we can learn to look for the truth of love, for the lesson that is made just for us. We can practice seeking out love in challenging situations and in difficult people, and the veils of disunity will show themselves. From there, we can work on clearing them.

This takes time, patience, falling, dusting yourself off, and going at it again. In practicing finding love, we're practicing seeing ourselves clearly. Through this act, we change our neurobiology. We rewire neural networks from our habitual shortcuts that promote separation, to a new way of experiencing ourselves and others: a connectivity, a compassion, a kindness, a learning. We re-create ourselves, and the rest of our lives follow suit.

Through this work, one thing becomes clear: ourselves. We become aware of incredible powers that lie, often dormant, within us—the power of forgiveness, resilience, softening, allowing, and breathing deeply. The power of faith and grace: grace, the strength to plant another seed; faith, the belief that it isn't all in vain. The yogic *Sūtras* remind us that it's when we see who we truly are, when we recognize our capacity to hold these virtues despite our flaws, and awaken to the fullness of our messy humanity and our extraordinary ability to contain it all, that we abide in yoga—in unity with ourselves and our environment. In seeing ourselves clearly, we see everything else with the same clarity. In this transcendent unity, love abounds; it becomes the only applicable truth.

This is how yoga saved my life. It became my greatest teacher through showing me that life is in constant communication with me, through the people I meet and the challenges I face. It saved my life by shifting my awareness from control to curiosity, from *Why is this happening to me?* to *What is here, right now, and how am I responding?* It has taught me to run toward my shadows instead of away from them, and to bring with me the torch of my awareness and love. The torch is the fire of seeking, meaning-making, and always finding that in every person and situation before me is a lesson. In each one of these, there is always something I can say *thank you* for, even if it takes me a little while (or years) to find it. Until I do, I trust, because the practice has never let me down. It has only ever met me and opened my eyes to exactly where I am at any given moment, which is right here, right now. And that's the only place I ever need to be.

PART II

The Practice of Yoga

19
GRACE, A SINGLE STEP

When on the day of my massive breakdown I was hospitalized at Bellevue Psychiatric, weighing slightly over eighty pounds, I couldn't remember the last time I'd eaten a meal. It had been months since I'd gone more than forty-eight hours without a panic attack, without fearing for my sanity. Anything was better than this. It was as though my will to live had slowly drained from me with every cut, and with time I could do nothing but shrivel up in the fetal position on my bed in my little room in Bushwick, Brooklyn.

During this time, I couldn't see outside my personal darkness. I couldn't understand why things had happened or why they still haunted me after years. Nor could I fathom any way out of the mess I was in. I couldn't imagine mustering the strength it would require to rebuild everything that had collapsed. I also couldn't picture continuing to live in fear of another impending panic attack, always looming around the corner; or live with flashbacks of death, abuse, and sexual assault playing in my head like strobe lights you can't unplug, like a bad acid trip you can't will yourself sober from. It was sheer madness, pure torture.

On my third day at Bellevue, one of the nurses called me into the common area. Vannesa had flown in from California. Her eyes were soft and swollen with worry, her little face so much like mine. She was pale and looked like she hadn't slept in days. She lit up the second she saw me, and ran to me immediately. She hugged and squeezed me the way Mami did when I was a little girl, when I'd wake up in the middle of the night with sweats from a terrible nightmare about ghosts haunting our closets.

I hadn't seen Vannesa in almost a year, and I'd forgotten the way her hair smelled like home, like family, like that one place where you can rest your head and the world takes on a softer quality. "I'm sorry," I whispered. Tears covered my face. "I'm *so* sorry." My little sister shushed me and rocked me and put her hand on my head. No one in my family and none of my old friends back in California knew how bad it had gotten, how low I'd fallen. Vannesa was the only one who came close to understanding how it could have possibly come to this. She was the only person I didn't have to explain anything to, the only one who'd seen it all with me, who understood the underlying sense of abandonment that had faithfully tagged along for most of our lives.

As soon as I saw her, and as she held me, I realized that she was the reason I couldn't give up, and that I did, in fact, have something to live for. Sometimes, we need those reminders, things we should have known all along; then, there they are, right in front of us, so clear. We held each other a little longer, two tiny orphans on a psychiatric ward in the center of New York City on a chilly autumn day.

Before my eventual release, I received an EKG. The panic attacks brought on heart palpitations, and the medical staff wanted to make sure everything checked out before I was let go. The results were normal, and as the cardiologist unplugged me from the machine she asked me if I'd ever taken a yoga class. I told her I'd taken yoga for two years in college and, even now, I did yoga from time to time at a gym in Union Square.

"I love it, actually," I said.

"But have you ever *practiced* yoga?" she inquired.

When I asked her what she meant, she replied, "Do it every day. Try it for a month. What do you have to lose?"

The beauty of hitting rock bottom lies in the realization that you've already lost everything anyway. It's in that surrender that grace arrives, though she's not infrequently fashionably late. In fact, we never really know when exactly she'll make her appearance. Grace comes when the spirit moves her. Anne Lamott talks about the messiness of grace, about how it's not an *abracadabra* kind of moment, but rather a sloppy and human thing. Grace happens … eventually, she says. Then, we can take the next step. That's what grace is: the energy mustered to take the next step.

We can take that step wobbling like a curious and precarious toddler, or like a toddler throwing a temper tantrum—kicking and screaming. Or we can take that step with a smile, try to dance along even if we're only pretending we know the song. But it's all different faces of the same grace. As we become softer and more delicate, more easeful and less resistant, as we practice falling and getting back up again, we realize that it's in losing everything that we stand to gain the most. We see that it's in the darkest hour that the dimmest light is most profoundly felt. And we're so grateful, even for the smallest of things. That's grace in all her glory.

A shaman once told me that the next step is the only step we ever need to take. And it's true. In fact, it's when we try to move ten steps ahead that we fall flat on our faces and are humbled by life. Grace in our darkest moments comes sooner or later, but I think her arrival is somewhat related to trusting that she *will* eventually arrive, in all her disheveled—*our* disheveled—glory: the brilliant muck of being wholly and blatantly human.

20
LITTLE STEPS INTO PRACTICE

My healing journey has not been elegant. Yet it has been filled with precisely what I believe grace actually is: clumsy little steps, with a fair amount of tumbling and bruising. I'm still an absolute klutz. It hasn't been quick, either; it hasn't been one of those awakenings you read about in books on Zen Buddhism—the sudden enlightenment brought on by a *koan*, like realizing that the sound of one hand clapping is a green bullfrog and *Bam!* the veil is lifted: you're a fully realized being. Not. Even. Close.

My healing has been slow and methodical; filled with pills and tears, relapses, re-cutting, and hating myself; moving forward with doubt, confusion, and plenty of frustration. I would say that today my path is *still* like this. I still consider myself an addict to OCD, self-injury, and anorexia, though recovering and about ten years sober. It's still messy, challenging, and confusing, and even triggering, only to a lesser degree. It's manageable now, and even enjoyable. There's a light in my path these days that I couldn't perceive before, and now I have a discernable guide I can turn to for straightforward and legitimate answers. This has made all the difference in the world: I found my *practice*.

I met Jhon only a few days after my release from the hospital. I had decided to commit myself to this yoga thing, because, as the cardiologist had said, I had nothing to lose. I spoke to my favorite gym yoga teacher, a woman whose class commanded a palpable respect and who knew exactly what she was doing. She told me about *her* teacher and said I should meet him, so I agreed.

At his yoga studio, Jhon greeted me and asked me to come into his office. He asked me about myself and I told him with trepidation, being sure not to disclose too much. I didn't share the gory details of my personal history or my recent hospital release. He listened and then asked me to stand up, to walk across the room and back, and then to simply stand. He studied my body and its movement and carefully watched my every step. He circled me and began to list the misalignments in my posture.

"Your inner arches are collapsed. Your knees cave in; they hyperextend and close your hips off. Your shoulders slant forward and when you talk you cover your chest with your right hand. You are hurt and you have not found who you are. You live in fear. You are lost." He ran through each point as though he were reading a grocery list, completely detached from judgment: these things simply *were*, and he was right about every single one. I hadn't even noticed that during the whole time I'd talked about myself I was hunching over and my hand covered my chest. It was as though I was protecting something sacred and defenseless. I stood a little taller and unbuckled my knees.

"If you want to get better, you need practice," he said in his thick accent. There was a clarity in his eyes I'd never quite seen in someone else.

"I have no money," I said. "I'm a student. I wanted to know if you offer any sort of discou—"

"I didn't say anything about money," he interrupted. "Do you want to practice?"

I did.

"If you commit yourself to coming here to study every day for one year, that is all the payment I ask for. It will come back around."

Jhon and I fulfilled our agreement. I became one of his most loyal students, coming to practice even when I didn't want to. I came if it rained or snowed or if the sun was shining and I wanted a break. I came if I had a cold or my body was sore or if I had research to do for my thesis. I studied with him every single day.

Jhon would say to me, "Tatiana, pick up your inner arches. That is your past collapsing your body. Pay attention. Wake up!" I never thought that my fallen arches related to my life, that my feet gave away how much of my past I was carrying with me, in my very muscle tissue. But he was right.

The more I practiced, the more I came to see that my body was like a map of my life and of my consciousness. I'd never realized that the two were, in fact, related; that they were one—no foreground, no background. The more I focused on creating an arch in my feet, on consciously lifting the roots of my body, the more I strengthened the muscles of my feet. My knees followed: the less they collapsed inward, the more my hips and spine came into alignment; the more my sternum rose and my chest opened, the less my shoulders hunched and the more I held my head a little higher. The more aware I felt in my body, the less I feared the world or my past because I could feel myself here, on solid ground. The more I learned about my body, the more insights I had about events that had brought me to where I was.

I was starting to cultivate a relationship with the body that had undergone such pains, both physical and sexual abuse inflicted by others, and the injury I'd caused it through cutting, starving, and loathing it. In the throes of my anxiety and panic disorder, the underlying theme had been that I couldn't feel my body. I felt as though I were hovering above it, unable to control it. In the middle of my panic attacks, I consistently felt as though I were dying, when in fact I wasn't. When they ended, the residual feeling toward my body was that it had tricked me. How, then, could I trust my body to know anything when it continually told me that something was wrong when in fact it wasn't? Not trusting my own body had been terrifying.

Now, I was learning the simplest of things. Jhon taught me how to breathe, how to stand, how to move slowly and mindfully, and how to inhabit the very vessel I felt so disconnected from for so long. The more I grew in my embodiment, the less afraid I became. However, the most important thing Jhon taught me was how to be still. "A posture means nothing without stillness," he'd say aphoristically. "You move too much getting in. Get in, then stop. Find the quiet in the pose. Then ease comes." In the stillness, in the struggle to find ease and in the noise to find that evanescent quiet, I learned that my emotions did not in fact define me, and that I was not my trauma. "Take a look," he'd say. "Watch the mind. Watch the body. What do you see?"

I spent many of our practice sessions in tears, unable to understand why meditation and yoga brought up more sadness in me. Hadn't I had enough? But the tears came and came, and Jhon said, "Let it be. Your job is to watch." In fact, when I first started with him, I wasn't able to close my eyes during meditation. Every attempt to meditate would send me into flashbacks that triggered my anxiety. "Open your eyes," he'd say, "and focus on a single point. Breathe. Study the breath." Years later I came to find out that this was a common condition for survivors of trauma and PTSD. Little by little, by returning again and again to my mat and my meditation cushion, my body began to recognize that this was a safe space for me to be in, and that I no longer needed to be hypervigilant. I still remember the first time I closed my eyes in meditation and saw... nothing. It was incredible—glorious, even.

On my mat, on my meditation seat, I cried for quite some time. However, my tears began to take on a qualitatively different feeling. I wasn't desperate; I wasn't reaching out for answers about the injustice of the world and the unfairness of my predicament. In this space, the question *why* simply didn't pertain. Something else was happening: the tears were *just tears*. It was as though I was taking care of a bodily function. It was as though I'd filled a jug with too much water and simply needed to empty it a bit so I could continue carrying it, function more efficiently, and be on my way. Jhon never hugged or consoled me. He never told me I was going to be okay. He never even asked me what was wrong. He didn't give me advice, either. To this day, I don't know whether Jhon knows much about my personal story. Jhon simply sat quietly with me and witnessed the sadness, the tears, the heaving, and, through that, taught me to do the same.

The process was slow: two steps forward, one step back. Sometimes, I took three or four steps back before another step forward. But one thing was true: the practice always, invariably and undeniably, showed me what the next step was, and my trust that that was the only thing I ever needed to know began to increase. I started to let go of the need to discover some eventual outcome. Instead, I focused on the patterns in front of my eyes. When I practiced, I felt clearer. I felt guided and less alone. I breathed easier.

Also, there were real-world, tangible payoffs. One noticeable and huge difference was the decrease in the occurrence of panic attacks. I remember the moment I realized that it had been two months since my last panic attack. I don't know if I was more in shock at that fact or by the fact that I hadn't noticed, which meant that my normative way of being, my natural level of anxiety, had shifted. I no longer expected fear as an integral part of my day-to-day experience. I wasn't sitting around consumed by anxiety, waiting for the next attack, the next hospitalization. My nervous system was beginning to heal. That alone was immense growth.

Not victimized by my own mind, by the threat of the loss of control, I started to feel more grounded and secure in a very foundational way. After a year under Jhon's tutelage, I was off all medications—antianxiety, antidepressants, painkillers, the cornucopia of bottles and pills that once sat in the palm of my hand. During the worst of it, I was taking seven pills, three times a day. I actually thought that this would be my daily routine forever.

My reintroduction to a social life proved to be more challenging. On the mat, I was learning control of my body and my breath, and in my sitting practice I was beginning to understand the contours of my mind, the things that made me tick, my triggers. But studies on a controlled and sequestered subject are radically different from taking methodology into the field. Add the unpredictability of other people, add *dating*—with its potential for disappointment and heartbreak on a heart that's barely beginning to mend—and that was a whole other endeavor (and perhaps a whole other book!). In dating I found myself re-creating familiar patterns from my youth. I found myself feeling like a victim again and very afraid; that provoked more tears and a sense of being out of control . . . and panic attacks.

I went four years without cutting and relapsed after a particularly difficult breakup. Stuck in a momentary hell of abandonment, I shredded my arms with X-Acto blades one especially snowy winter. Only this time it felt different: it wasn't the same high, the same release. This time I didn't just cut: *I watched myself cut*, which was qualitatively different. It felt toxic. It didn't work anymore. And that was the truest of all changes— that I could identify toxicity and feel it as *undesirable*.

I was no longer the same. This time, I fully recognized my old patterns. I realized I was re-inviting thoughts and sentiments of fear, loneliness, and abandonment, and bore witness to it as it all transpired, rather than doing so months or years later. Even if I got caught in suffering, a great shift within me had already taken place, and it had changed everything.

Every relapse, whether physical or mental, was also different in one crucial way: I had a place to return to—my practice. Recently, I was telling a friend about how I learned to swim. I was four years old and my parents enrolled me in a class. On the first day, the instructor was giving the class a tour of the pool and, mid-sentence, out of nowhere, he pushed me into the deep end. Having never been submerged and with nobody in the pool to help me, I panicked. Then, I heard "the rope!" and through my blurry, stinging eyes I saw a rope about a foot away from me. Some sort of innate survival instinct took over. The next thing I knew, I was clinging to the rope and pulling myself to the edge of the pool.

To me, it's as simple as this: life without practice is life without a rope. No matter how deep the pool—the sorrow, fear, anxiety, sense of abandonment, or any other of the very human challenges that we're bound to experience in this beautiful, messy experiment we call life—you won't drown if you have your rope.

It's been over a decade since I first met Jhon and he introduced me to what has become one of the greatest gifts I've received in my life: my practice. He was right about many things, including that it all comes around. After my apprenticeship with him, I volunteered at his studio for several years, and now teach philosophy trainings and seminars for aspiring teachers there. Over the years, I've had the opportunity to work with hundreds of students, many of whom remind me of my old self: hunched shoulders, shattered hearts. Today, I can see in their bodies what Jhon saw in mine, and I can hold that same space he once held for me. As a result, I've had the immense privilege to watch earnest, young yogis blossom into self-inquiry, and start to settle into their budding practices.

Since my first days with Jhon, my practice has shifted and deepened considerably, and I expect it will continue to do so as my understanding continues to mature and I immerse myself in the awe of recognizing that the more we know the more we realize we really don't know much at all—then softening into that space of uncertainty. There are still the simple things, which are ultimately the most profound of all. Today, I love those things that once ailed me most. That doesn't mean that I don't struggle; it means that I've learned to find (or at least search for) the stillness and ease in the pose of being with each of my struggles. It means I've learned to relate to them in a different way, to communicate with the struggle as I might have with my parents, if they were still here. I've learned to ask the struggle to be my teacher, and to do my work of recognizing the barriers within me that are keeping me from coming into any situation with anything less than an open and accepting heart.

Today, I love my mind: the same mind I feared to be left alone with and that replayed images of past horrors on repeat for years. I've learned that this very mind can also replay wonders—that for all the things it's forsaken, it can also find blessings and miracles even in the murkiest of places. I love my wounds. I love their depth and all the effort, work, and sacrifice it's taken to heal them: the countless hours on a mat, in meditation, in prayer, in journaling, in a self-discovery so vast its endlessness both envelops and soothes me.

I love that because of my wounds I've had the opportunity to work with victims of domestic violence, with women who were self-injurious and suicidal, and even with their abusers, and that I've had the opportunity to create a safe space for that vast array of experiences. I love my mind and my wounded/healing heart because I can talk to abusers and somehow connect to their humanness, to *their* wounds, to the degree of lost-ness and darkness that it requires to hurt another person out of your own hurt. I love my mind because it allowed me to find humanity in the claws of brutality, and that's how healing is born for each one of us.

I also love my body in a way I never imagined I could. I love it with all its flaws and imperfections and perhaps *because* of all its flaws—its hundreds of cutting scars like pins on a military lapel. I love that my obsession with controlling my body flourished into a lifelong love affair with the human form, anatomy, and the way that bones stack on bones and muscles, ligaments, and fascia, bringing them all together. I love learning and teaching how to properly care for this wondrous biological system, this miraculous machine, so that we may feel brighter, lighter, and more in tune to its messages. I love that my body, which was once my enemy, is now my best friend, and better yet, one of my great teachers. My body has become a guide to my life itself: to my work with others, to my relationships, and a vital key to my spirituality.

I didn't learn or love any of this all at once. It was step by tiny, awkward, scary step.

21
THE ELEMENTS OF PRACTICE

In Part I, I presented an account of the basic philosophical tenets of yoga, alongside a very personal account that I hope illustrated the pertinence and impact of their application. As I've indicated on more than one occasion, I believe that yoga saved my life, and it's for this reason I've felt compelled to share the power of this practice in my writing as well as in my teaching on and off the mat.

Throughout, I've alluded to "the practice" of yoga and "the work" of yoga. However, I've barely scratched the surface on the specifics of what constitutes a "practice," and what, exactly, "the work" entails. In the following chapters, I provide a more detailed, pragmatic "how-to" application of the theory. Many of the exercises I describe aren't drawn strictly from ancient yogic texts. Instead, they're practices that have been passed down to me through several teachers, many from different lineages, and some I've developed on my own. They all have one aim: the cultivation of awareness that shows us the road home, back to the presence of our hearts.

After presenting the theory of what yoga is and how it works in his first book of the *Yoga Sūtras*, Patañjali also becomes practical. As Swami Satchidananda (one of Patañjali's translators) points out, "Mere philosophy will not satisfy us. We cannot reach the goal by words alone. Without practice, nothing can be achieved."[24] Similarly, Pattabhi Jois, one of the greatest teachers of yoga responsible for bringing and growing yoga in the West, was notable for saying, "Practice, practice, and all is coming."[25] Ultimately, practice is the backbone of philosophy; otherwise, philosophy becomes just a theoretical nicety.

For this reason, Patañjali's second book of the *Sūtras* relates strictly to the yoga of practice—yoga in action—and in it he lists several tools for practice, a number of which we'll examine here. Toward the end of the list, Patañjali closes by saying, "Or any [tool] one finds uplifting may be used."[26] Yoga is not prescriptive in a *thou shalt do this or punishment will be cast down on you* sort of way. In this practice, there is no means–ends scenario, nor the threat of hell. We create our own punishment, for no external circumstance can compare with the power of our internal demons. The opposite is also true: complete freedom and authentic joy spring not from external wealth but from internal clarity. It's the state of our inner landscape—the strength, maturity, openness, and softness of our hearts—that determines the peace we feel at any given moment, especially in the most difficult moments.

Let's be clear here: the path of yoga is a training, and a very particular type of training at that. It is interested in self-inquiry, learning, curiosity, and ultimately the exploration of questions: What if we could come to anything at all—any situation, person, or pain—and not be shaken, but instead be truly ready for what it has to offer us? What if we could cultivate a heart and mind capable of being with it all? The answer to these questions can't be articulated; it can only be experienced. The answer is the quality of our lives themselves. These are not easy questions, nor is this an easy path.

The path of yoga necessitates dedication and perseverance. Dedication and perseverance constitute, in fact, a second meaning of the term *tapaḥ*, which I used in Part I. *Tapaḥ*, or self-discipline, is the word that opens the second book of the *Sūtras*. The second word is *svādhyāya*, or self-study.[27] It requires equal parts fierceness and softness to cultivate the type of heart that can grieve without losing its center and love without expecting—a heart that can be open to whatever arises, capable and ready to withstand everything. It takes resolve to free ourselves from decades of conditioning and courage to explore the ways in which we are conditioned. It needs fortitude to look deep inside ourselves with curiosity instead of criticism and ask, *What is* really *going on here right now?* It necessitates strength and time to cultivate the patience and hone the craft of listening enough to be able to sit and hear a response, and then to develop the tenacity to say *yes* to whatever that answer is. Yet, above all else, this path requires practice.

Any artist from any discipline will tell you that their art is as much, if not more, a development of proficiency in a set of skills than a reliance on creativity or talent. The painter is truly a painter when painting is her way of life; the same is true for the writer—the writer writes whether he wants to or not, for he knows that it's not about his eloquence but the placing of words on the page that ultimately matters. For all their inherent talent, professional athletes gain high degrees of dexterity in their sport through rigorous training, many of them since childhood. The yogini who can balance on her forearms and bring her toes to touch her head in the most perfect of scorpion poses has practiced that *āsana* thousands of times. There are no shortcuts: the groundwork of mastery *is* practice. Practice, practice, and all is coming.

"Success in mastery," Patañjali's *Sūtras* say, "depends on whether the practice is mild, medium or intense."[28] Later, Patañjali observes: "Gradually, one's mastery extends from the primal atom to the greatest magnitude."[29] No value judgment is meant here; we are free to choose the degree to which we wish to attain mastery in anything. True mastery occurs when the object of our mastery becomes our way of life. The object of our focused attention is that which grows most, and we have full choice on what that focus becomes.

In the yogic path, practice is a lifestyle. This is to say that if our object of mastery is yoga (union, right-seeing, joy, peace, freedom), then we aim to imbue our lives with the practice of these principles. It is then that practice transforms from something we "try to get in when we have the time" or something we "do," to something that's integrated into the very structure of how we go about life itself. In other words, an integrated practice of yoga ultimately changes our relationship to life itself, where every moment becomes an opportunity to practice and the process fills us with curiosity, clarity, and joy.

22

MAKING LIFE A PRACTICE

Laozi (Lao Tzu), the author of the *Daodejing* (*Tao Te Ching*), warned wisely: "Don't think you can attain total awareness without proper discipline and practice. This is egomania."[30] Lasting change usually doesn't occur overnight. Although it's possible to experience powerful epiphanies or moments of enlightenment (many of them coming from often surprising and even tragic life-altering events), and they may instantly change the way we see our lives, the change in consciousness we seek is most often cultivated gradually. Lasting change requires time and sustainability.

Consider, for example, losing weight. Most of us give up on diets because they don't work; simple fixes aren't really fixes because after we've lost our weight, we go back to our old ways and fall back into pre-existing patterns. Diets are, by definition, temporary in nature. The work of yoga isn't a consciousness diet. For change to take hold it requires that we make a commitment to adopt a whole new paradigm. Further, it needs the change we create to be sustainable and manageable so we don't give up two weeks in. To this aim, it's helpful to remember there is no race, no rush. Instead, ours is a gradual opening into presence that expands who we are so radically that we can permanently shift the quality of our lives.

As we experience the qualitative alterations in our experience, the work becomes softer, and often, more enjoyable. We also don't need to know where we're headed. As we wake up, the next steps tend to reveal themselves, so long as we're ready to pay attention. Once we take that step, the following one becomes clear. The degree of our practice will also change and transform our relationship to our current work and to what that work reveals for us. A commitment to a five-minute meditation may feel incredibly hard. However, if you stick to it, gradually (or suddenly), you may crave twenty to thirty minutes a day of that same stillness. Mythologist and historian Joseph Campbell once pointed out that when Jesus said to his disciples "My yoke is easy," he meant, "My yoga is easy." As we grow in authenticity and union with the crux of who we are, the practices that cultivate that awareness become second nature. Our yokes become easy.

Initially, however, change requires concerted effort. The walls of conditioning we've built around ourselves are often reinforced by years of steel-like thought patterns. As we develop in practice, however, and dismantle our walls, the process eases. Surely, there are waves of intensity in the work; at times, we can even feel overwhelmed. The *Sūtras* list some of the obstacles and accompanying hardships that we may stumble on: "Illness, negligence, misperception, dullness, laziness, failure, doubt, craving, instability, mental and physical pain, unsteadiness in the body, sadness and frustration, irregular breathing," to name a few. Yet the *Sūtras* also provide the way out of these troubles: "The practice of concentration on a single subject or the use of techniques is the best way to prevent the obstacles and their accompaniments."[31] This is our antidote.

Even in the most challenging of times, say as newbies struggling to establish our practice or as seasoned yogis moving through different layers of subtlety within the practice, the path helps us keep going. Through beautiful, scattered moments of bliss we gain insight into something new: be it realizing that eating bread before bed is keeping us up at night, or that a certain friendship is toxic, or simply that we slouch and that's the source of our indigestion. Whatever it is, the insight arrives with an uplift, a greater vision, an understanding. These are not only valuable and meaningful events—they also *feel* amazing. So, we come back, and we remember why we are here, doing the work.

Until our practice becomes easy—or rather, until we learn to infuse our practice with increasing moments of ease—it is helpful and important to create structure around practice. Several *sūtras* are devoted to the notion of practice itself, and they're worth exploring here. It's normal that in any path we choose to take we'll find challenges that can leave us wondering, *Am I doing this for nothing?* or *Where are the fruits of my labor?* Yogic philosophy outlines three elements that act as cornerstones to the concept of practice that help us touch base with where we are. This is the definition of a firmly established practice as provided by the *Sūtras*.[32]

I. A Practice Is Done for a Long Time

In the grand scheme of things, practicing for three years isn't a very long time. Imagine that your practice is a child, and imagine the insight, wisdom, and understanding that you have at age three. They would be very different from those of a fifteen-year-old. That maturity continues into the late twenties, and deepens further in the thirties and forties, as it solidifies into a truly rooted maturation. The longer we practice, the more we gain from it. In moments of doubt and frustration, it's helpful to remember the age of our practice.

2. A Practice Is Attended to with Consistency

When one learns anything—to read, write, draw, do handstands—mastering that practice is directly proportional to the consistency and depth of the time and rigor spent in that practice. This is to say there's a big difference between drawing once every few months and committing oneself to draw ten minutes a day, every day. Clearly, the person who devotes him- or herself to drawing every day for an hour will develop the ability to draw at a different rate than the person who does so once a month for five minutes. Studies have demonstrated that mastery of complex tasks is gained after 10,000 to 50,000 hours of practice.

Nike got it right with their slogan, JUST DO IT, and that's my biggest piece of advice here. Understanding the inner workings of the philosophy of yoga, its relevance to our lives, and its capacity to profoundly heal our wounded hearts all depends on a commitment to consistent practice, which can prove challenging to sustain.

In all fairness, practicing daily can sometimes feel outright boring. I can think of a million excuses to skip my practice this day, or this week. However, these are *precisely* the moments when our practice can teach us most about our minds—the way they function and the way we find refuge in things that perhaps don't serve us. In terms of practice, one of the most valuable gems is that practice as such is really a relationship with effort; we move through effort to come to ease. Ease, however, isn't static. We gradually grow toward easefulness through a play with effort and struggle, which return when they have something to teach us, and light up the places where we find our work cut out for us.

The analogy of a garden comes to mind here again. If our mind is a garden, and the healing of our hearts is akin to the garden blooming with the most exquisite of flowers, then the *vṛittis*, the movements of the mind that are ultimately made up of our *samskāras* (our unhealed wounds that for years have constructed our view of our lives), are the weeds and pests that threaten the health of our flowers. Anyone who's gardened knows that the work is ongoing; once the flowers have bloomed, they must be kept healthy and alive. Even if the weeds are removed, their roots can re-emerge if we assume that we no longer need to dig them up. And then there's always the next season.

3. A Practice Must Be Attended to in All Earnestness

The third and final element of practice is purely internal. There's a qualitative difference between accidentally stepping on a person's toes and doing so on purpose. Even though the physical event remains the same, the intentionality behind it changes the quality of the event. This quality is internal in nature. Likewise, the amount of earnestness we give to our practice has an influence on the result of our efforts. Given that we're embarking on a lifelong journey of healing and self-realization, we cannot expect growth to flower from half-hearted efforts. Through time, with consistency, and by giving it our all, our efforts pay off. As the *Bhagavad Gītā* reminds and encourages us, "On this path, no effort is wasted, no gain is ever reversed; even a little of this practice will shelter you from great sorrow."

23
TAKE THESE FIVE PRACTICES

To create lasting change in our lives, we must have an anchor. As the *Daodejing* points out, practice is our rock, our steadiness; it is what grounds us in our growth. Without practice we can't expect change nor can we measure our growth. Hence, the next question that arises: If the yogic path is about making our lives themselves a practice of unity, awareness, joy, and love, then what can we practically do to accomplish that?

Rumi wisely asks us to consider, "Do you make regular visits to yourself?" The *Sūtras* make the same call, reminding us that the way in is always through ourselves, here, now. *Svādhyāya* (self-inquiry, study, and reflection) is the crux of this work, and the *Sūtras* provide a sampling of specific practices that aid us in the process of honing our concentration and paving the road to self-study (some variations of which I provide in the following pages). Yet one of my favorite *sūtras* reads: "Or [disturbances of the mind are cleared] by meditating on anything one chooses that is elevating."[33] This means that we can choose whatever methods most call to our hearts in order to learn to cultivate our focus. Each person has a distinct way of connecting with his or her own path, and sometimes the work becomes finding out what tool fits best where we are, at any given moment.

I believe that, even in our most muddled moments, we always know exactly what we need to do, if we could learn to listen to the intuitive wisdom of our bodies and hearts. All we might need is a little push, or a reminder or suggestion to get us on our way. In fact, I'd wager that you already knew a substantial portion of the philosophical exposition in these pages, just perhaps not in these exact words. The truth has always been there. Yet occasionally we need a clear strategy or a direct approach.

In the Workbook are what I call "The Five Practices." They are:

1. Practice the Witness
2. Practice Allowing
3. Practice the Shadow
4. Practice Greater Mind
5. Practice Surrender

These practices are structured after predominant themes in the *Sūtras*, and like the *Sūtras*, each practice moves from the gross, physical, or tangible to the subtler. Although these practices work on the premise and the work of the practice before it, the road to healing and awareness isn't necessarily direct; our lives, as our consciousnesses, are creative and nonlinear. Therefore, although I encourage you to read them in order, I trust that the ordering of the practice will become your own as you take it on.

Many of these exercises can be used either when life brings up a particular event or as a means to cultivate a structured, daily routine. For the latter, I find that early morning, lunchtime, or evening are good times to incorporate practice. You can carve out anywhere from five minutes to an hour for this work, depending on what you're working with, where your practice is at that time, and what you feel you need. You can also practice at different times. If you know you're very busy on the weekdays, you can create a short five- to fifteen-minute weekday practice, and then set aside half an hour to two hours of practice time on the weekends. The flexibility here is endless, and the more you practice, the more clearly these elements will reveal themselves. The practice will speak to you and to your needs—at times softly, at other times as loud as an alarm clock whose snooze button you keep wanting to hit. However, the practice does develop a voice; all you have to do is pay attention and heed its call.

An additional suggestion is to keep a practice journal. This, too, will inevitably become your own creation and method. However, one way to start is simply to write down what and when you're practicing and any insights that might have come. For example:

I sat and counted my breaths, focusing on lengthening and expanding my breath while paying attention to the reactions in my body. I did this for fifteen minutes. I realized that I hold a lot of tension in my lower back and that it probably has to do with the way I sit when I work.

Additionally, many of the exercises I present below come with journaling reflections or questions that can further the work of the exercise. The journaling can become its own practice, as some people find great release and reflection from writing. At the very least, journaling serves as a marker for accountability, and a method of keeping track of what's worked, when. I've found that for me, exercises that haven't "worked" or that haven't seemed to fit my life at a certain point were later extremely useful at another point in my life. Sometimes, it's simply about where we happen to be at any given time, and what speaks to us at that moment.

You can never grow out of these exercises; in this case, practice doesn't make perfect! As you find your own style, you learn to hone and move with what makes sense for you, and the practice becomes yours. These practices are mere suggestions, a way to kick-start you on your path, or to help in times when you feel stuck. At its heart, the connection to ourselves is creative, flowing, and spirit-like; the structure that consistent practice provides is the yang to the yin of fluidity. Creating strong channels in our practice is what allows the waters of our creativity to course with both ease and direction. Structure and flow are as symbiotic as they are integral to developing strength and accessing the softness of our healing hearts.

Further, my experience is that some people get turned off by philosophy and awareness exercises when they are to be performed in the solitude of one's own space. I've found practice on my meditation cushion, in the privacy of my inner self, to be absolutely essential for its application elsewhere in my life. However, I recognize that some want their exercises in an applicable context "off the mat," if you will. In moments when my own practice is lackluster, I think of things that inspire me: the yogi who can effortlessly float into a handstand; how writers I admire make words dance gracefully on the page. I know that for each of these seemingly effortless accomplishments, hours upon hours of private drilling and practice have taken place: our private practice is the behinds-the-scenes work that makes the play on stage come to life. That said, the best (albeit more intense) practice may require jumping into the deep end. In our context, this is our practice in the world—with real people, in real-time situations.

The greatest marker of our inner growth is not how many hours we can sit motionless on the meditation cushion. It's how often we smile; how much we care; and how much love, kindness, joy, and presence we bring to the people and situations that cross our path. For this reason, I've included specific "off the mat" versions of exercises titled *Applied Practice*, in addition to the more traditional *Home Practice* exercises.

Finally, let me mention that the exercises may initially feel a little long, arduous, or self-evident. To this, my analogy is explaining to someone the step-by-step procedure for tying shoelaces. If you were to write it out, it would make the process seem complicated, especially if you took the time to distinguish between the different approaches (i.e., bunny ears vs. loop around), and go into the detail of each. Yet, we all know that after a little bit of practice, tying shoelaces becomes second nature and doesn't take long to perform. The same principle applies here: it takes longer to write and detail the exercises below. In reality, with time, the exercises become your own and almost instinctual. So, once again, I invite you: *Ehipassiko*—come and see for yourself.

The practices I share in the Workbook are very close to my heart. They've guided me in times of sorrow, confusion, and fear as well as joy, peace, and gratefulness—and continue to do so. One of my teachers once said, "Things work until they no longer work." Although I provide several different exercises that can help us remember who we really are so we may be those mirrors for one another, not every exercise will work for every person all the time. That's the fun of this path: the exploration; the ability to take something, play with it, make it your own, discard it when it no longer serves, or pass it on when it does. It keeps us on our toes. I hope you do all of those things and perhaps more with these exercises—all an amalgam of my years of study in academia, on the mat, in the classroom, in waking life, on my meditation cushion, on my knees in prayer, in the fetal position when I couldn't find the light, and through writing—when my practice gave me the strength I needed to put my fingers on the keyboard, tell my story, and write this book.

In the (many) moments where I doubted the practice and questioned the value of the work, I often came back to some of my favorite words from Anthony de Mello,[34] which so beautifully encapsulate why we embark on this inner journey:

"Is there anything I can do to make myself Enlightened?"
"As little as you can do to make the sun rise in the morning."
"Then of what use are the spiritual exercises you prescribe?"
"To make sure you are not asleep when the sun begins to rise."

Namaste.

WORKBOOK

The Five Practices

WITH ACCOMPANYING EXERCISES

Contents

IV. Practice Greater Mind

V. Practice Surrender

I

PRACTICE THE WITNESS

I described practicing the witness in Part I. Witnessing is the most fundamental of all yogic and awareness practices. Indeed, if you had to choose a single practice to stick to, this is it. Witnessing is the ability to pause at any moment and step back from your immediate experience to create a space of observation. From this place we watch, take note, and learn.

What exactly are we watching? One theme that appears throughout the *sūtras* is that of working from the gross to the subtle. We begin with the obvious and tangible and slowly work inward, to the places that are slightly more challenging to perceive, which are often the most powerful. The exercises on witnessing work in this progression, starting with the physical body and moving inward. ■

Exercise I
Witnessing the Physical Body and Establishing a Baseline

Home Practice

Developing a structured practice, ascertaining a baseline of where our physical body is, and creating a space and peace within are the central practices and foundation for our work as they deepen and increase in subtlety. The body is a beautiful instrument that is always present to guide us and tune us to its wisdom, as well as to teach us to mediate its reactions.

This practice begins with establishing a baseline and noticing where we are at any given moment. This may simply mean seeing where our bodily and mental tension is. Are we usually relaxed, maybe even slightly apathetic, or do we struggle with being high-strung? Do most challenges feel surmountable or like emergencies? Witnessing where we naturally tend to "hang out" along the spectrum of tension and stress is not only an important tool but one that registers shifts with time and practice.

Establishing a baseline requires continual practice, ideally every day or every other day, and maybe several times a day for shorter intervals. Continuity is perhaps the most integral aspect of practice. Humans are hardwired for habit; we just need to learn to choose those habits that serve us best. To establish continuity in practice, choose a practice time that's reasonable—as short as three minutes or as long as an hour, depending on the structure of your days. How long is not as important as continuity. Choose a time you can commit to on a daily/semi-daily basis without it feeling overwhelming. After deciding on a time of day, choose a place. The ideal space has minimal distractions, where you can sit in stillness without disruption. Once you've chosen a time and space, you can begin.

Come to your space and take a comfortable seat that supports your back but still allows you to sit upright and alert. Don't lay on your back if you can avoid it; it's easy to lose focus and fall asleep. Once in an upright, comfortable, supported seat, close your eyes or soften your gaze on a single, unmoving object about a foot in front of you. A candle or a familiar object can be nice. Deepen the breath. Take five to ten breaths, noticing the cooling inhalations as they enter the nose and the warmer exhalations as they exit through the nostrils.

After five to ten deep breaths, scan the body and notice your state of mind. On a scale of one to ten, rate the degree of tension, with one being a feeling of complete stillness, aware relaxation, and the ability to breathe without many interrupting thoughts and ten being a huge struggle to sit still, complete physical discomfort, and thoughts that race so much it feels torturous simply to remain seated. Take note of the number.

When conducting your tension inventory, you can break the body into segments: the feet and legs; the thighs, abdomen, and buttocks; the chest, arms, and head. Provide each section of the body with a number pertaining to its degree of tension. To scan the mind, count an additional five to ten breaths and notice the frequency and urgency of interrupting thoughts, and also give the mental disruption a number.

Take at least another five breaths before ending the exercise. Try not to judge the number but utilize it simply as data—useful scientific information without positive or negative associations. Write the date and number(s) in a journal, and repeat the following day.

A shortened version of this exercise can be done for one- to three-minute intervals throughout the day: in the morning, midday, and before bed. Journal your findings. After a week, you can ask yourself and respond in your journal:

- What patterns came up?
- Are there correlations between the time of day and the activities that take place during that time and the degree of physical or mental stress/discomfort you experience?
- Have the numbers changed as you've continued the exercise for several weeks?

After several weeks, you may have more access to a baseline, which then allows for more exploration and experimentation:

- What daily occurrences seem to increase the number? What activities decrease it?
- Which occurrences can you increase or decrease to gain more relaxation through the day?

Journal your thoughts and observations as you move through the exercises and notice as patterns reveal themselves. ∎

An Important Note on Trauma

For some who've experienced deep traumas, the simple practice of sitting and closing the eyes might not be appropriate. If closing your eyes during these exercises is triggering or creates flashbacks, conduct the exercises with your eyes open. If sitting in stillness with your eyes open is also triggering, please consult a licensed mental health professional.

Exercise 2
Witnessing the Physical Body and Introducing Stressors

Home Practice

Something I find very special about this work is that the more we practice, the better we get at it. This is especially fascinating when working with the physical body. As we tune our instruments of perception, we become more aware of what our body needs, and more capable of taking care of those needs. These are just some natural and positive byproducts of our work in witnessing.

Learning to read our bodies begins by listening to them, paying close attention to sensations, and noticing the shifts or movements of those sensations. When we become acquainted with bodily sensations while the body is at ease, say in seated meditation, we can also learn to pick up more efficiently on its cues when our body isn't centered. As we've established, suffering, unease, sadness, and heart wounds ultimately live in and are perpetuated by the mind. Yet, each emotional state has a physiological counterpart. When we're sad, we often place our hands on our chests; when we're afraid, our shoulders tense up, and so on. We may not even realize that we aren't well or know what is "off" until we check in with our bodies. It's then that we can identify what's really happening.

Just like the body can be a map to what's going on within us, it can guide us *out of* the funky places, especially when we find ourselves in a rut. Although the mind can easily wander into the past and jump into the future, the body is always squarely grounded in the here and now. The body is a perfect landing space to return to when we realize we've mentally left our center and perhaps tumbled into a vortex that doesn't serve us. For this reason, practices designed to raise awareness of our physicality like *haṭha yoga, taiji (tai chi), qigong (chi kung)*, and to a degree even running and sports can be powerful tools as we undertake internal work. This is perhaps why in the West the word *yoga* has become associated with the practice of *haṭha yoga/āsana*, or postures. These exercises, when executed correctly, are themselves a training in mindfulness and presence that tune us to our bodies.

Honing in on the language of our body, we can learn to use the body as a map to navigate the difficult moments. We can decipher the language our body speaks through witnessing and observing sensations in our physical bodies in different situations.

Body-Scanning

Home Practice

Find a comfortable seat where you feel supported in your spine and back, and tall and alert. You can close your eyes or soften your gaze on a single, unmoving object about a foot and a half in front of you, so that visual stimulus isn't distracting. Take five to ten deep, slow breaths so you can arrive in your seat and fall into your body. Imagine that with each exhalation, you're releasing any cluttering thoughts or any activity from the day so far (or the day ahead), and you're finding more space in your mental landscape. Close your eyes if you haven't done so after your ten or so breaths and bring to mind something you associate with peace. It could be a scene by the side of a lake, or your grandparents' porch where you spent your summers as a child. It can be someone whose presence puts you at ease, or a word or an abstract idea. You could even simply repeat the word *peace* in your mind.

After you feel settled in this space, scan your body. Witness where your mind goes first:

- Your feet?
- Your belly?
- Your chest?
- Your head?

Take note, but do nothing. Continue scanning and notice how comfortable you feel:

- Where do you feel most at ease?
- What part of the body has easily surrendered?
- What part of the body do you barely feel because it's so quiet, almost imperceptible?

If there are any areas of immediate tension, simply breathe into them until you feel an overall relaxation. This can last anywhere from five to thirty minutes. Then, bring to mind something slightly uncomfortable—something small, like a spat with a sibling or coworker over something petty. Now notice the body:

- Where did the mind go immediately?
- What has shifted, and how?
- Was there a body part, external (your shoulder, leg) or internal (your stomach, liver, kidneys, lungs), that your mind went to immediately?

Note the involuntary physical reaction and where it took place in your body. Take a few moments to breathe and return to the space of calmness, to clear the stressful thought with ten or so more deep breaths. Thank your body for allowing you to work and learn from it, and don't exit the exercise until you can tap into the ease you had before inviting the uncomfortable experience.

Through the experiment, we learn about the shifting bodily sensations that can occur as a result of a negative thought or memory. Some people will feel constriction in the chest, others might feel heat in the stomach area, and still others might feel intensity in the throat. Our body is a guide to our emotions, and our emotions are a guide to the playground our minds are frolicking in and the mental friendships we're keeping. Thoughts have the power to shift our physical sensations, and hence our ease at any moment, just like shifting our physical sensations through gaining a calming breath can affect the thoughts that we—perhaps inadvertently—are choosing.

This simple body-scanning exercise brings to light the synergistic relationship between bodily sensations and emotional stressors. Through this exercise we can learn how our particular body reacts to manageable emotional distress and our specific correlations in the physical body, which may be a key to where we hold stress. We can take this useful information with us into our physical practices, like stretching or yoga, and pay special attention to those places that carry the physical load of our emotional stress. Simultaneously, we can pick up on the power of redirecting our awareness toward our breath as a way to ameliorate the buildup of tension created by negative thoughts.

Secondly, gaining awareness to how our body processes challenges can provide us with valuable information about how to shift *out of* difficult moments. When we understand our body is aware and awake to the present, and that a symbiotic relationship exists among our body's sensations, our thoughts, and our experiences, we're more easily able to shift how we respond at a time when it might be beneficial or necessary to do so—such as in real, waking life.

Applied Practice

Applied practice pertains to how we apply the tools we've acquired to daily life, often in interactions with others. At the end of the day, we are relational beings that exist within a context and not a vacuum. Applied practice helps us notice our patterns as they relate to the influence that others have on us, and helps us to mediate our reactions so we can turn them into aware and intelligent responses. In so doing, we foster growth in our interactions and relationships.

No relationship is without its difficult moments. Yet these have the capacity to become some of our greatest teachers. However, it's critical we possess the specific tools to handle and learn from difficult moments instead of becoming enmeshed and caught up in the reactivity they tend to elicit. Learning from challenges is a conscious choice we make at every moment, but we have to first recognize what the lesson is. Pausing to witness the physical body during an intense experience, discomfort in a conversation, or difficult interaction can be extraordinarily revelatory, and the number one means of avoiding saying or doing something that might cause more harm than healing to someone else or to ourselves.

For applied practice, it's good to start with a moment of slight discomfort, something that arises out of a benign conversation. Most days, something small will rub us the wrong way and we can shrug it off. Without replying or planning a response, and without doing anything at all, simply pause and notice:

- What changed in the body?
- If you had to name a particular body part that it affected, what would it be and how was it affected?
- Was there a tightening, a heating up, a cooling off, a rising, a falling?

Becoming aware and identifying the quality of the shifts in our bodily sensations during uncomfortable moments can teach us how our physical body responds to conflict, disappointment, sadness, surprise—any emotion. Hence, we not only gain greater insight into our reactive mechanisms but also into what physical sensations are linked with what emotional states. Ultimately, we can discern what thought patterns and even what words and actions are our weapons and our crutches in times of stress.

Creating awareness by simply noticing our bodily sensations during a difficult moment instantaneously shifts how we relate to the situation as it transpires. In this shift, we're automatically choosing a different lens through which to look at it and cultivating a nonreactive response. We become curious about our own experience and settle there before moving forward. When we become familiar with the subtleties of our patterned reaction responses—which can take place in a fraction of a second—we can learn how they function, so we can ultimately shift them altogether. Through this work, the space between our stressor and our reaction grows, and, in that space, choice arises. In focusing our awareness on the body, we immediately change our relationship to what is occurring as it's happening. ■

Exercise 3
Witnessing the Breath

The breath is one of our sharpest teachers. The breath is sometimes an automatic response to what we're thinking, and hence how we're feeling. Learning to become intimate with our breath can take us beyond the turnings of the mind and into the simplest of truths. The breath is also the ultimate metaphor for the movement of life itself: it comes and it goes, and we need both in equal proportion. When the breath stops, it becomes uncomfortable. If we hold it all in, we eventually have to let go, and we can only be completely empty for so long until we eventually have to let some breath in.

Humans are mammals with automatic breathing (meaning we don't have to think in order to breathe), unlike other mammals, such as the dolphin, for which every breath is a conscious choice. Because our breath is something that can go unmonitored without causing us harm (we could, theoretically speaking, live out our entire lives without ever thinking about how we are breathing), we tend to take the breath for granted, and in doing so, we miss out on its role as a powerful tool and teacher. The breath is in fact so powerful that the word for breath in Sanskrit is *prāna*, which translates as "life force" or "vital energy." And it's true in the most basic sense: Without breath, we don't have life. Therefore, it follows that in learning to alter the breath, we learn to alter the force in our body, and hence, affect our experience palpably.

Through witnessing the breath we can learn volumes about ourselves. The breath is key to our emotional state. In fact, the two go hand in hand. Deep emotional responses all have corresponding breathing patterns: When we're startled, we hold our breath; when we're sobbing, the breath is heaving and gasping; when we're laughing uproariously, we're also looking to find our breath; and in times of anger, the pragmatic advice is to take a few deep breaths and count to ten.

We also know that when the mind is at ease, the breath is also calm. The relationship between the breath and the mind is as complementary as it is dynamic. This is to say that when we shift one, the other one is also affected. We find, though, that between the mind and the breath, the latter is the easiest to change voluntarily. It's far more accessible to bring awareness to our breath in order to change it (i.e., take a few deep breaths when we realize we're holding it) than it is to change our emotions at will (it's far more difficult to shift extemporaneously from sadness to happiness). The breath is our key to learning how to voluntarily adjust our mind-states.

Breath Counting

Home Practice

The most basic of home practice exercises is to establish a regular practice of sitting and watching the breath. Begin by finding a comfortable, upright seat, where the spine is supported. Observe how you feel, and without modifying the breath, pay attention to your breathing pattern. Allow your mind to wander for a controlled amount of time—two to three minutes. Notice if the mind wanders into stressful territory, and if it does, check in on the breath and register changes.

After a few moments of allowing yourself to remain in unrestrained breath and thought, bring it all back to controlled breathing and mental focus. Return your awareness to controlled breaths and count ten to twenty rounds of breath, equalizing and elongating the inhalations and exhalations. Count out the length of each breath, and see if you can make the next one slightly longer, until both are at about an even six to eight counts long. At the end of the breathing exercise, notice how you feel and take note of the qualitative difference. Journal your findings.

Full Breath, Empty Breath

Home Practice

Spend a few moments settling into a comfortable and supported upright seat. Take a few cleansing inhalations and exhalations, and when you feel ready, inhale slowly and deeply. Count the length of your inhalation until you feel you can no longer take in any more air, and hold. Then, sip a little bit more breath and hold. Try taking one last sip of air. Hold the in-breath for as long as you're able, and pay attention to the thoughts that arise and the level of discomfort that comes up for you in mind and body. When you need to release the breath, do so in a slow and controlled fashion. Take a few deep breaths to center yourself, and repeat the exercise. This second time, hold on the exhalation. Release as much breath from your body as you possibly can, then a little more, and hold. Once again, bring awareness to the thoughts and feelings that arise at the sensation of complete emptiness, and when you're ready, breathe in slowly. Finish the exercise by taking a few rounds of normalizing breaths, in and out.

You may take a few moments for reflection and/or journaling and consider the following questions:

- On a scale of one to ten, how uncomfortable was it to hold breath in?
- What thoughts/emotions came up while you held your breath in?
- Did any memories come up as you held your breath?
- How did you feel when you finally exhaled?
- On a scale of one to ten, how uncomfortable was it to hold the breath out?
- What thoughts/emotions came up while you held on empty?
- Did any memories come up as you held on empty?
- How did you feel when you finally inhaled?

Notice which of the two was more or less comfortable. It might be worth considering that the level of comfort/discomfort with holding breath in is related to how easily we're able to receive. Conversely, the level of comfort/discomfort with holding the breath out is related to how easily we're able to give. Additionally, we might note the memories, thoughts, or images that came to mind at the height of discomfort in each in- or out-holding experience and reflect on whether these relate to things in our life we're holding on to, or things we're not allowing ourselves to receive.

Shift in Breath with Added Stressors

Applied Practice

The applied breath-work practice is as simple as witnessing any shifts in our breathing patterns during uncomfortable moments in our daily interactions. It's easier to notice that something has shifted if we're already familiar with our baseline. The same principle applies here as well: the more we strengthen our home practice, the more effective our applied practice tends to become. In home practice we're truly developing self-knowledge; in applied practice we're introducing variables.

Becoming aware of how the breath changes during uncomfortable situations, like a conversation that took a negative turn, or sitting in traffic, or perhaps even at a boring board meeting, can provide us with a lot of information. Any of these situations can be stressors; more than likely, the stress will be reflected in our body's reaction and will be clearly felt through changes in our breathing.

The first part of the applied practice is to notice. Keeping a journal of simple notes can be very helpful for establishing patterns. It can look something like this:

Stressful activity:_____ (e.g., work meeting, argument with my partner, stuck in traffic)

I noticed my breath:_____ (e.g., breathing fast, holding my breath, breath felt struck in my throat)

Corresponding emotion: _____ (e.g., frustration, anger, sadness)

By journaling our breath patterns alongside stressful activities and corresponding emotional states, the patterns of how our own particular system—nervous system, emotional system, respiratory system—works will become clear. Once we have this insight, once we've lit up these unconscious patterns with consciousness, we'll be more likely to effect change in our experience, by effecting change in the breath.

Breath Work in Real Time

Applied Practice

After establishing our patterns, or once we feel comfortable with our baseline patterns of breath and emotion, a second applied practice is to use the breath as a tool to shift ourselves out of reactive emotions. As with all of our applied practices, we begin with something small. Through our journaling exercises, we can look for patterns and pick a certain activity that seems to consistently elicit a stressful emotional response and a corresponding ragged breathing pattern. Choose an activity. For our example, we will use sitting in traffic.

Begin by witnessing and watching the breath change and the emotion (let's say, frustration) arise. Then focus on the breath exclusively. Let the emotion be, and instead shift the awareness to the breath. Effect change on the breath, and bring awareness to it. As in our home practice, allow the breath to take up a greater area of your awareness. One strategy is to simply count the length of the breath in and the length out. At the sign of an interrupting thought, acknowledge the thought, and then return to the counting as an anchor, and see if the breaths can be lengthened to a count of eight. Do this for several minutes, and witness any changes in the stress levels.

In the event that the stressor occurs in the middle of a conversation, the technique is simply to notice the breath when the mind runs into reactivity. You may notice one before the other, but simply take note. It may be difficult to count breaths if you're in the middle of an argument, for example. If it's possible to take a break from the argument, to step aside and breathe, then consider doing so. If not, then simply noticing the breath in the middle of the situation will be enough to bring some awareness to the automatic stress responses. Once the interaction has ended, you can resume the exercise, taking time to count out the breath.

Journal your findings. Here are some questions to consider as you write:

- If you were to rate the level of emotion on a scale of one to ten (with one being not stressful at all and ten being extremely stressful), where was the stress level at the beginning of the exercise?
- Where was it after breaths were counted and lengthened?
- How difficult was it to return the awareness to the breath?

- How powerful was the pull of the interrupting thoughts?
- As the breath lengthened, how did sensations in the body change?
- How did the emotion change? ∎

Exercise 4
Witnessing Language

The *Sūtras* ask us to pay close attention to the words we speak. The second book of the *Sūtras* suggests that we take note of the degree of harm or aggression (or lack thereof, *āhimsa*) and truth (*satya*) in our speech. Our words are non-physical actions fully capable of creating physical consequences. They're also a key to the realm of our thoughts, even the unexplored crevices of our minds.

Because the key to witnessing our language is to pay attention to our unconscious patterns, the practice of noticing our language is most effective in the applied setting, as we are relating with others. One of the most helpful exercises in observing language I've found is choosing a focus each day, week, or month, and journaling our findings.

Witnessing Our Words

Applied Practice

Choose a focus that you'll commit to monitoring in your verbal interactions for a set period of time (one day, three days, a week, a month), and commit to a journaling schedule so you can count the uses of your set focus for that time period. The journaling could be as simple as opening a note-taking app on a phone, and simply keeping count of how many times you employ the focus you've chosen.

Here are some examples of foci you can choose and note:

- How many times you speak negatively about yourself
- The types of words you use to describe yourself
- How many times you apologize out of habit (for profuse apologizers)
- How many times you interrupt another person when they're speaking
- How many times you speak negatively about another person

- The types of words you use to describe other people
- How many times you speak with the intention to hurt, put down, or criticize another person
- When you don't say what you mean
- How many times you speak negatively about a situation
- The types of negative "predictions" you make about a situation that hasn't yet happened
- When you use passive-aggressive language or tones
- When you're being purposely unclear
- How many white lies you tell
- How many full-on lies you tell
- How many times you use words that immediately or later make you feel uncomfortable/negatively/regretful

The list is endless and adaptable to the patterns you already know you have or suspect you might have. Again, keep in mind that the first step to any change is simple observation; bringing awareness to the words we say can shed light on feelings we may not even know we have. All of this is good data to add to our findings of self-discovery.

Witnessing Words Around Us

Applied Practice

As we explored in Part I, we humans are deeply contextual beings. The background of our lives (our relationships; the spaces we inhabit to live, work, and relax; the media we consume) has a deep influence on our experience. In truth, there's no foreground or background—it's simply a matter of perspective. All experience is happening simultaneously, and we tend to frame the subtle aspects of our lives as backdrops to our primary actions, goals, and achievements. For this reason, we may be less likely to notice the subtler aspects of our environment unless we really pay attention, and as we already know, the subtle can be revelatory. Hence, practice and training suggest we pay attention to our surroundings, which undoubtedly play a role in structuring our consciousness, even when we don't notice them.

In the applied practice of witnessing words, we can start by noting instances of overtly negative messages that surround us every day. Listen to the words spoken by those on the train, on the bus, in the office, in the media you consume, and in the music you listen to or overhear as you visit a store/coffee shop/or other place you may regularly attend. For this exercise, pay attention to and count and journal how many times overtly negative messages appear in your environment during a set period of time (an hour, day, or week). Note the following:

- Were there any patterns?
- Were there particular words, phrases, or themes that occurred within a particular context (i.e., phrases, words, or themes that continually popped up in music, or in the speech of friends, family, or coworkers)?
- To get even subtler, what is the general mood that occurs within each of your spaces? What is the body language of those around you?
- By paying close attention to these, did you notice any sensations in your own body and/or energy levels?
- After the set amount of time (an hour, day, or week) are you surprised by your findings?

I can offer one very clear, brief example from my personal experience. I noticed I was feeling drained and generally down at the end of the days when I traveled to teach. I paid attention to the words, body language, and general energy of my day and found that my commute felt very stressful. To reach my destination quicker, I tended to take the express subway train, which was without fail packed with people in a huge rush, many of them not acting their friendliest. Every time I got onto the subway car, it felt like a fight and a struggle. Once I recognized the ride itself was a stressor, I tried a different route—on the local train, which most of the time was almost empty, and the ride was more calm. This route took twenty minutes longer, yet I noticed I felt more relaxed and had more energy for the rest of my day. Therefore, although taking the local train has added an extra eighty-minute commute to my week, it's become an oasis for me, a time to reflect without worrying about the phone calls, text messages, or emails I have to tend to. It's a time when I read or listen to an uplifting lecture; it's one of the moments I most look forward to in my week.

In this example, my environment played a major role in how I felt, and therefore, how I was likely to act toward those around me. Taking the time to pay attention, notice patterns, and journal our findings of the ways in which our environment affects us allows us to take action and limit what we expose ourselves to. In this way, we create subtle change in ourselves.

Another way we can realign our context is to pay attention to the messages from the media and our surroundings, depending on how we're already feeling. Many of us relate to certain types of music, talk shows, magazines, and conversations when we're already feeling out of balance. We can pay attention to our environment during different moods and emotions and consider the following:

- *What is the prominent mood/emotion: Sadness? Fear? Happiness? Distrust? Anger?*
- Do you choose a particular medium when feeling this way (e.g., playing sad love songs when you feel unhappy, playing angry music when you feel irate, or listening to talk shows that are aggressive in nature when you feel similarly)?
- What are the recurring words/ideas in these media?
- Do you turn to particular friends or conversations, and if so, do they tend to reflect the same emotion you currently inhabit?

As we've explored, much of our human conditioning is geared to re-inflicting our wounds. It's almost as though we believe we might not be able to feel any longer if they healed. One way we preserve our hurt is by stimulating that same emotion within our environment. If we feel heartbroken, we may listen to songs about heartbreak; if we feel preoccupied with some aspect of our physicality, say our weight, we may surround ourselves with media that accentuate ideal (yet impossible) body types, thereby keeping us (and encouraging us to remain) within the energy of the negative emotion.

Which comes first—a negative feeling we have or the surroundings that either spawned it or perpetuate it—may be unresolvable. However, it's clear our emotions and surroundings are intertwined. Understanding this about ourselves, we can move into awareness, which is the seed from which lasting change grows. ∎

Exercise 5
Witnessing Thoughts—Patterns and Stories

As we move from the gross to the subtle, we arrive at the most nuanced realm: the thoughts. Establishing a witnessing practice with our language can open a great doorway into the mind. With its infinite plasticity and flexibility, the mind can be our dearest friend or most treacherous enemy, and its contents determine the quality of our lives. We've seen what's at stake; it's the very stuff of yoga: stepping into our inherent connectedness and inborn goodness, our ability to be and love and laugh and let go, enjoy, and welcome life as it unfolds. Witnessing in the mind is the first step away from our tendency to be careless with the mind. Don't be careless with the mind! Instead, be gentle and soft with, and curious about, what lies inside.

In a class I led recently, one participant, a young woman I've known for several years, cried as she shared how scared she was to meditate. She was afraid of watching her mind. This isn't an uncommon response. When we're honest with ourselves, many of us, I think, fear what beasts are prowling in the crevices of our mental darkness.

We'll never know until we observe. That exploration doesn't have to be profound and intense at first. Depth will come when the time is right. For the beginning student of the practice of observing, the focus remains on creating and cultivating a steady, consistent practice. In this case, that means watching the thoughts and thought patterns, and using the breath as an anchor for the present moment, where we're safe and secure. As the work solidifies, the next, perhaps deeper or subtler, steps will reveal themselves. I touch on the deeper work in later chapters.

Who Do We Hang Out With?

Applied Practice

We begin with applied practice, because unexplored patterns tend to reveal themselves most in our daily lives. Start the day with an intention to observe your mental friends. Personify your thoughts, and think of them as folks you hang out with that serve you, or friends that don't—as if you're back on the playground in middle school with the kids who were trying to convince you to skip class or get into some other type of trouble. If thoughts are your friends, then who are you hanging out with for most of the day?

It's easy to forget our intention as we get caught up in our daily tasks. We can use the tools at our disposal to cultivate the qualities we're working on. One trick is to set an alarm for every three or four hours that simply says, *Pay Attention*. At each interval, we can inventory the predominant thought patterns that have risen over the past few hours. We can write them down in our mindfulness journal. For instance, in the last few hours, did you experience any of the following:

- Get caught in any thought trance/vortex?
- If so, what was the predominant theme?
- Did you project negatively onto a person or situation?
- Did you leap into the future about a situation you currently have no control over?
- Were the feelings associated with it predominantly negative or positive?
- Did you look into the past, replaying conversations or situations in your head?
- Were the feelings associated with it predominantly negative or positive?
- If you spent a lot of time in a vortex of future or past, was there a triggering event/conversation/activity that led you downward?

Becoming aware of where we tend to hang out mentally is easier when we take inventory at regular intervals. We're more likely to forget if we wait until the end of the day and try to remember what tripped us up. Likewise, we're more likely to catch ourselves in our recurring and often unconscious patterns if we set an alarm rather than wait to do it all at once. Both techniques help us be accurate and honest with ourselves.

If we get caught in a negative thought-trance, notice the sensations in the body and the emotional states that come along with them. It's likely that those negative mental spaces, our schoolyard frenemies, are encouraging our perception of separation and alienation, and keeping us trapped in a particular story that we keep unconsciously perpetuating, and hence projecting and re-creating. The mantra here is *Pay Attention*. Notice. Write it down. Repeat.

The Stories We Tell

Home Practice

We may have a fairly clear idea of what the daily thought-traps that keep us feeling separated are. We may know that if a certain song plays it will remind us of a negative experience that will trigger memories and projections. We know that if we hear a certain name, or walk through a certain part of town, our minds will take over. If we're aware of such triggers and of the direction of our thoughts, then it's time to explore a little further.

With your journal at hand, find a comfortable seated position. Settle the body and mind using your favorite breathing technique. After anywhere from three to twenty minutes of breathing and settling, choose a thought pattern you know you have. Begin with one that isn't loaded or that doesn't have a lot of trauma attached to it. Maybe it's a breakup that annoys you, and when you think about it you get stuck and feel irritated, rather than one that breaks you down. Always start simply. Tell yourself the story of what happened as if you were narrating it to someone else. Simultaneously, listen to the story you're telling as if you're hearing it from someone else.

As you're telling/hearing the story, identify the thought patterns associated with it:

- Do you repeat past experiences but digress to discuss different possible outcomes?
- Do you wish you'd acted differently?
- Do you project into the future?

Pay attention. Now ask:

- Where in the story do you feel small and separated?
- Where in the story do you feel disconnected and triggered?
- What are the feelings?
- Where are they in the body?
- Is there a sense of loss of control and disempowerment? Victimization?

Establish a basic outline of the story, and find the underlying theme. Journal your findings. Much of the time, triggering events that lead us into mental trances are those that arouse feelings of disempowerment within us. Although there are certainly situations where our options are taken away, the fact we're reflecting on these events is proof we have options here and now. It's common for our sense of disempowerment to carry over into our lives, and to seep into our ideas about ourselves. In so doing, we can make choices that support this feeling; we re-create situations similar to the ones that originally hurt us.

Paying attention to the story at hand, try to boil it down to a simple thematic sentence: *I am always left behind*, or *The lucky things never happen to me*, or *I'm always betrayed*, or *I'm not good enough*, or *I always lose*. Take this theme and look for other stories in your life that leave you with a similar feeling. For example, in my life I noticed that I felt I was consistently being taken advantage of at work: *I always work hard but my efforts aren't noticed, and my bosses take advantage of my goodness*. It happened over and over again, for many years. I wasn't earning what I thought I should earn; I was doing more work than I originally signed up for; when I moved to a different position, the pattern continued to reemerge. Until I worked with it.

Identify and journal the pattern. Now ask:

- What am I doing in my life to reinforce that pattern?
- What are the thoughts associated with that pattern?

Consider:

- If life is ultimately infinitely interpretable, there's a possibility I'm interpreting my choicelessness and my victimhood. Is there another way this story can read?
- What can I do to change the narrative?

Pay closer attention to the stories you tell yourself, especially those *about* yourself. That is your homework. Watch, journal, repeat.

Pervasiveness

Applied Practice

Pick a time that you'd like to practice observing pervasiveness: a day, week, or month. Observing pervasiveness in our thought patterns requires becoming mindful of our mode of operation during challenges that arise.

When a challenging situation with potential for a negative or positive outcome arises, what is the pervasive response? Pay attention first to the bodily sensations. The act of noticing will itself create space. Notice without responding:

- Does it feel like your body is under attack and you want to attack back? Is there aggression?
- Do you feel overwhelmed and wish you could run away and hide?
- Or do you feel you must defend your ground?

Then pay attention to what happens mentally:

- Are you more likely to assume/fantasize/play out the negative or positive outcome?
- Which of these feels more likely: the negative or positive outcome?

Say that the negative outcome plays out, or you are given bad news about a situation:

- Do negative outcomes feel like they happen more often? Do you think something along the lines of, *Of course this would happen*?
- Or do negative outcomes feel more like an anomaly, just bad luck this one time?

Say that the positive outcome plays out, or you are given good news about a situation:

- Do positive outcomes feel like they happen more often? Do you think something along the lines of, *Of course this would happen—it's what I expected all along*?
- Or do positive outcomes feel more like an anomaly, just good luck this one time, and you can hardly believe it happened?

Through witnessing, we can familiarize ourselves with our degree of pessimism versus our degree of optimism. The pessimist is more likely to interpret negative outcomes as routine and positive outcomes as anomalies; the optimist will see positive events as the natural flow of life and negative ones as anomalies. You can ask yourself and journal:

- Where am I in the spectrum?
- What is my first assumption when something negative happens?
- What is my first assumption when something positive happens?

As we've already seen, our perspective is everything. The yogic path is partially teaching us to unlearn our mental habits, so we can inhabit a space of peace. We find peace, partially, by recognizing that every event in our lives, every situation—no matter how personal, positive, or negative it may seem—is ultimately value-neutral. The yogic work teaches us to hone the tool of the mind, responsible for how we experience our reality. Although we have full control of this perceptive tool, it works mostly on patterning, and it's this very patterning that determines our experience. Hence, it behooves us to recognize that we are deeply responsible for our perceptions, and to take on the work with the patterns: to commit ourselves to understanding them and to molding them in such a way that they bring more peace into our lives. It's necessary for us to be the guardians of our own minds, to stand awake and aware at the doorway of our own consciousness, and be mindful and selective of what or who we allow to enter.

Although the *Sūtras* have been describing our abilities to change our mental patterning for thousands of years, it's only more recently that Western science has found that, in fact, the brain has what we now have come to understand as neuroplasticity. In other words, the brain is malleable, and we can consciously effect changes in our brain function. With practice, we're able to create new neural networks that amount to new patterns in our perceptions, and even our immediate reactions. This means that positivity, happiness, joy, peace, and even love are all *practices*—and they all require training, repetition, and time.

It all begins with that first step: witnessing. Once we pay attention and take the seat of the witness, our perspective has already undergone a shift. The rest is practice, practice, and more practice. So, if you've noticed throughout the above exercise that you feel predisposed to a negative pattern, you can practice changing that perspective. You can ask yourself these two questions:

- What if the outcome isn't negative?
- What if I imagine the best possible outcome in the situation in front of me? What change might transpire then?

Journal, and find out. ∎

| |

PRACTICE ALLOWING

The practice of allowing asks us to spend time with whatever we've witnessed, and let it exist as it is without our input. In truth, much of our yogic practice is training to permit ourselves to embrace the wholeness of what's present, both externally and internally. As we grow in our practice of allowing, the barriers to allowing that exist within us reveal themselves, providing us with valuable insight into what keeps us bound, whether it's to current situations that don't work for us or grievances and emotions we've been carrying with us for ages. A substantial aspect of practicing allowing is learning to see and remove that which keeps us from growth, and ultimately from the freedom of a liberated heart.

As we touched on in Part I, there are three main places where we can work on allowing: with others, in life situations, and within ourselves. ■

Practice Allowing with Others

One of the best areas for growth is our relationships. No relationship is without its days—or even seasons—of challenge. If it's a meaningful relationship, difficult moments with the ones we love can suck energy from us. When we aren't in a good place with a partner, sibling, parent, or dear friend, that malaise can seep into other parts of our lives, making it difficult for us to concentrate and easy for us to obsess about the problem or argument.

The foundation of allowing with others rests on a basic premise: We're all equal, and we're all walking the same path to self-discovery. Though our roads may look different and our timelines might be dissimilar, one person's experience is as important as anyone else's. As we go through our own journey, it's easy to become entranced by our own particular story and undermine that of others. We fail to see them as equal and their story as valid as our own. Allowing others is about waking up to our radical equality, and learning to lessen our expectations regarding another's path. In doing this, we arrive at compassion—not only for others, but for ourselves.

Exercise I: Creating an Internal Freedom Landscape

Home Practice

For this practice, keep your journal at hand. Start in a normal meditative and alert position. Take five to fifteen minutes to calm your breath with exercises like counting the breath or listening to a serene piece of music that will leave you in a balanced place. Once you feel settled, bring to mind a situation with another person that is bothering you. As usual, it's helpful to start with something small and move deeper with practice. Bring to mind the elements of the disagreement or stalemate, and then take a look at your position. Notice:

- What happens in your body?
- What are the thoughts and emotions that come up for you?

Let the mind wander into the "What if?" territory of your argument, of whatever place you are wanting the other person to change, and identify:

- What aspect of the person's behavior do you want to change and how?
- What are your concerns or fears associated with this? What if they don't change?
- How many of these fears pertain to the future?

Journal your responses. Remind yourself that the future doesn't exist. What exists is the present moment. Return to the moment at hand, and consider:

- From what positive place is this person's behavior right to them?
- What comes up for you in the sensation of wanting to change another person or their behavior?
- What does it feel like to want to change another person?

Usually, the sensations are uncomfortable. Consider:

- What would happen if you didn't want to change the other person?
- What would happen if you created space for them, and hence for yourself, here and now?

Recall that the essence of love is freedom and respecting freedom. This is as true for self-love as it is for loving another. Notice what is keeping you bound to the situation. Visualization can be extremely helpful here. See if you can get a visual image of what's binding you to the situation, and then imagine that dissolving. Imagine yourself and the person you wish to change in a growing space filled with light, compassion, and the best intentions. Bring to mind a serene, affirming, and open landscape. (You can each be in your own field of flowers, in the ocean, or at the beach; whatever is most pleasing to you.) Imagine space and openness. Imagine any negative links dissolving for you both. Imagine each of your paths trodden with understanding, discernment, and authentic action. Dwell in this space of visualizing openness for some time, and allow yourself to soak up your inherent freedom.

In this field of space you can notice the following:

- What feels different within me?
- In what way does the other person seem different?
- Am I more likely to tune in to their inherent goodness when I see them and recognize them in their freedom?

As you complete the exercise, notice differences in your body and mind. Do you feel less bound, less restricted, and more free?

Liberating ourselves from attachment to control is a practice like anything else, and it sometimes requires gentle reminders that we aren't the keeper of another's path. We can remind ourselves of this truth through meditation and visualization.

By creating freedom for ourselves and for others within the space of our minds, we're more apt to recall that inherent freedom in our interactions and hence more likely to appreciate, respect, and prioritize it in our relationships. When we experience freedom in our relationships, we're less likely to trigger reactive tendencies in each other or reopen old wounds. In allowing a space of freedom for another person, not only do we provide that same freedom to ourselves, but we say: *I accept you and I honor your freedom to choose your own path*. That is love in all its liberty.

Exercise 2: The Internal Landscape of Freedom in Real Time

Applied Practice

After we've practiced creating an internal landscape of freedom during home practice, it's far easier to bring that same quality of openness into our interactions with others. The same principles apply, though the process might be slightly different.

After spending some time in home practice, moments of discomfort or an impasse in an argument with another person will change their quality. You may notice (or bring to mind) first your experience in your body, which is always tethered to the present. If it's possible, take a break to breathe and pay attention to the signals your body is sending you. Perhaps by now you're more familiar with the physical sensations and mental stories that are linked to emotions of fear, anger, sadness, etc. Notice.

Now, identify the specific ways in which you want the other person to change. Observe any sensations of restriction you might experience and identify them, name them. Then, bring to mind the landscape of freedom for you both at that moment. Create that space internally, and know that you accept this person, their path, and their choices as they are now, and that you are consciously allowing both yourself and them the freedom to be as you and they are. You're allowing the experience to express itself as it needs to right now, as it's in your path perhaps to help you learn this very lesson. Breathe.

If you found it helpful to work with affirmations or statements, you might add, *I fully embrace your inherent freedom*. Relax your shoulders, hands, and facial muscles. Notice whether, as you relax and allow, the other person also relaxes. Perhaps they do the opposite: take the opportunity of your allowing energy (which they may or may not be consciously feeling) and use it to vent more. Allow the other person to undergo their process. Allow yourself yours (which may include separating yourself from the situation if it isn't safe for you physically or emotionally). Or perhaps you stay and witness the person as they are in their vulnerability. Breathe and hold the space for you both in your mental landscape. See what develops.

Our ability to hold space will expand with practice, and with practice it will become increasingly easier to witness and allow the physical sensations to dissipate and the attached mental stories to quell. You may want to take time afterward to journal:

- What was different in this interaction?
- How did you feel during the interaction?
- If you noticed mental distractors that tried to keep you from attaining that space, what were they? (This is good material for future introspection exercises.)
- What was it like to create a mental space for you both?
- Do you think the other person could feel the space you were creating?
- Did your feeling toward the other person or their choices change or transform as you invoked the freedom landscape?
- Was their attitude, approach, or behavior affected?
- Was there a different outcome?
- How did you feel after the interaction?
- What changed?

A Note on Allowing the Other

Allowing others is a technique for situations that meet the criteria of basic emotional and physical safety, love, and respect. It is sometimes difficult to tell whether a relationship is unhealthy, coercive, or abusive. I am in no way condoning allowing others to take away our most basic right to love and respect. In the event you need guidance navigating a potentially abusive relationship, please contact the National Domestic Violence Hotline for resources and expert help.

Exercise 3: Making Room for Listening

Home/Applied Practice

Philosopher and poet Mark Nepo says that to truly listen is to lean in with the willingness to be changed by what we hear. So often in our interactions with others we face barriers that keep us from being able to hear, and hence truly see, who they are. These barriers keep us locked into our own sense of identity, and in times of conflict they keep us fixed on our story, unable to fully grasp another's experience. We're often unwilling to listen fully because we might feel judged or misunderstood ourselves, or because we have an important point we want to get across, or because our environment isn't conducive to listening (we have the TV or a video game on; music might be playing; or our face is in the paper or a book while we nod, and "listen").

When we aren't completely present to listening, whether due to internal or external barriers, we miss out not only on the wholeness of those we are in relationship with but also on our own growth. We miss out on the ability to heal: ourselves, our relationships, and one another.

Recall the metaphor of the lake from Part I. We look into the lake and see our reflection (however distorted or clear it may be) and our entire environment in that same way. True listening is a way to clear our pond, or as Nepo says, to allow ourselves to be changed by what we hear. In true listening we consciously allow another person to be who they are and focus on the moment at hand. By doing this, we leave our habitual means–end paradigm and step into yoga. There, we become pliable.

True listening heals because at the very foundation of who we are is a wish to be seen and acknowledged. When we're in pain, distress, or another form of suffering, and another person can meet us in full presence, nothing else is necessary. No advice, suggestions, or tricks are necessary—just listening and being with.

Most of us have at times brimmed over with emotion, worry, or concern and had a friend listen to us as we vented. We gave our impassioned rants, and after some time, we ran out of steam, took a big breath, and let out a sigh. Without saying anything, our friend, by their presence and ability to hold space for us, allowed us to release whatever we needed to let go. This is healing. By the same token, I'm sure we've all experienced moments when we've had something on our minds or in our hearts and in the middle of sharing with someone we've discovered they aren't truly listening. This can be disheartening.

It's not difficult to tell when we have another's full, undivided attention, and when we don't. Nonetheless, providing another with our complete presence can be challenging. We can take a look at our own barriers to listening and maintaining presence by noticing both the external and internal obstacles we face.

Externally, we tend to be habituated to our environment, which may not be conducive to true listening. In this arena, all it takes is for us to create a space adequate for listening, where there are no distractions, such as television, music, or media of any sort. If we've been practicing sitting and witnessing, we've familiarized ourselves with silence already, and the task becomes easier. You can consider:

- What environmental distractors make it difficult for me to listen?
- What changes can I make in my home/office/space to make it easier for me to focus on the other person?
- If I'm speaking on the phone with someone I care about and they require my full presence, what activities am I simultaneously engaging in that are keeping me from being there?

The internal challenges are those that arise within us as we listen. We've all experienced these occasions. The best way to figure out what they are is to pay attention next time you're asked to listen, and see if any of these or other tendencies arise. You can make a checklist:

- How many times did you interrupt?
- How many times did you ask follow-up questions before the other person completed their original thought?
- How many times did you ask for clarification or elaboration?
- How many times did you catch yourself thinking about something else?
- Were you multitasking?

Additionally, it's worthwhile considering, and even journaling:

- What does it feel like to be heard?
- What does it feel like to *not* be heard?

Exercise 4: Co-listening

Applied Practice

The following exercise requires a partner. When practiced appropriately, this exercise provides a hands-on experience of the effects of true listening.

The exercise consists of each partner taking turns being the Listener and the Speaker. Once you've decided who'll be the Speaker first, designate a time frame. If you're playing with the exercise to get a feel for it, I suggest starting with three to five minutes for each role. If you're using this exercise as applied practice in a discussion where there's tension, you can spend as long as twenty minutes in each role. Once you've done the exercise several times, it will be easier for you to tell what allotted time makes the most sense.

The Speaker will begin by speaking nonstop for the allotted time—say, five minutes. The Speaker must speak for that entire time. The reason for this is that after some time, it will feel as though there isn't much more to say, but this is where we hit gold. If the Speaker continues to talk, they may discover some hidden, underlying emotions. During this time, the Listener does nothing but listen—no interacting, and no asking questions, even if they want clarification. They simply listen. At the end of the allotted time, the Listener reflects what the Speaker said in five or so bullet points. The Listener must avoid interpreting, commenting on, or responding to anything the Speaker said, and instead reflect what the latter said as closely as possible.

After the reflection, the parties switch roles and repeat the exercise. Both parties must agree to drop the conversation for at least twenty-four hours after the end of the exercise. By the end, both parties will have been heard, without an opportunity to react to one another.

Take some time to journal:

- What did it feel like to listen without being able to respond to the other person?
- What did it feel like to speak without being interrupted?
- What did it feel like to speak until the allotted time ran out?
- Did the listening or speaking section feel longer?
- What did it feel like to not have a back-and-forth discussion/argument?
- What did you learn about yourself as a listener?
- What did you learn about yourself as a speaker? ∎

Practice Allowing Situations

Most of us have experienced serious states of uncertainty, where we're waiting for an outcome that might involve a significant shift in our lives. We might be waiting to hear back about a job we've set our hearts on or an offer from an academic program; or an even higher-stakes scenario, such as the results of a medical exam.

These moments can be excruciating: the passing minutes can seem like hours, and days like weeks. They're moments when the world reminds us that we're not as in control as we occasionally allow ourselves to believe we are. In the practice of allowing situations, we let ourselves be humbled by the truth: we're just one part of a greater, continually developing picture. Our reaction to the waiting time not only creates the quality of our experience during that process but can also tell us a lot about where we stand in our ability to let things be as they are.

Allowing in the arena of situations is deeply intertwined with our ability to witness; only now we take it a step further.

Exercise 1: Tear It Up

Home Practice

Begin by creating a conscious, meditative space for yourself, where you can sit and reflect. Have your journal at hand. Start simply with a few minutes of breathing until you feel calm and at ease. Allow yourself to feel easeful in your body—in your facial muscles, throat, chest, and belly. Once you've reached a settled place, bring to mind a situation that is waiting to unfold (or you can employ this tool when a situation arises that requires you to wait it out). Hold it in your mind for a moment, and witness the changes in the body:

- What happens to the heart rate?
- What happens to other areas of the body: the face, throat, chest, stomach, hands, and feet?
- What has changed?

Now notice the subtler shifts:

- Are there words or stories that immediately arise?
- What expectations of the outcome are coming up?
- What expectation are you most attached to?
- What emotions does this cause to arise?

Take a moment to journal your findings. Include any reactions, fears, and even eagerly anticipated outcomes. Put yourself on the page. Then, rip the page out of the journal and tear it into little tiny pieces (or burn it in a safe environment). Notice what this feels like. Leave the torn (or burnt) pieces of paper and return to your seat. You may employ a mantra, affirmation, or repetition strategy:

I am here, now.
I am not bound to outcome.
For this moment, I am free from any results.
I allow my situation to unfold in freedom.

As we practice materializing and then destroying our expectations, often linked to negative emotions and anxieties about the future, we return to where we presently stand. It's from this space that we can access the most real thing of all: our hearts as they are now. The more mystical theories also suggest that when we expand our heart-space, this same space will be reflected outward, into the situation. In the end, we feel the release of the tight grasp the outcome has on us, and learn to allow ourselves to be more at peace where we are now.[35]

Exercise 2: Personify It

Home Practice

When we resist what is unfolding, we perpetuate the gap between the world as we think it should be and the world as it actually is. This is a space of separation, in which suffering abides. Healing begins when we stop resisting things as they are. Otherwise, we're caught up in an imaginary reality from which resolution cannot be born, since no problem can be solved from within the energy of the problem. We must first identify what internal reactions the external world is producing, and then create a space for the drama to play out.

I want to note here that the process of allowing in no way means we condone injustice, whether personal or social. I'd argue the opposite is the case: it behooves us to work toward a more equitable world. Yet, we can take actions from a segregated place within us, which are likely to be filled with negative, unchecked, reactivity or we can take them from our inherent wholeness. This is the work of allowing (and later, the work of the shadow): to integrate what we're not aware of, so our actions are clear and come from a place of integrity.

The process of allowing is primarily internal, but it requires us to abide, for some time, in a space of non-action until our internal lake is calm, and we've become clear.

For this exercise, in the comfort of your home, begin by taking your quiet, still, upright, and alert seat, and employ breathing exercises of choice to enter a place of relative relaxation. Pick a situation that's either currently unfolding or has already unfolded and that makes you slightly uneasy. Remember, it's easier to start at the shallow end; begin with situations that are slightly bothersome, rather than deep and painful. Eventually, with practice, these exercises can be applied to more complex situations as well; but it's helpful to get a feel for the work before diving into the deep end.

Once you've identified the situation, name it. Try to make it one word. It can be a name that makes sense, or one that pops into your mind. Now the situation is personified. Imagine that the situation has a form, some sort of a body.

- What does it look like?
- What does it sound like?
- Identify some of its traits. Allow it to speak. What does it say?

Now notice your reaction to the personified situation. What emotions arise? Pick one, two, or three. You'll work with each individually. Pick the most salient emotion, identify it as best you can, and repeat the process: name it and personify it.

- What does it look like?
- What does it sound like?
- Identify some of its traits. Ask it to speak. What does it say? Perhaps it tells you a story.
- What is this story, and is it a story from your life? A dream? A childhood fear?

Repeat the process for one or two more emotions. Now you have a small cast of characters, all with their own names and stories, and all with something to say. Notice which one creates the most visceral reaction, and where it rests in the body. Allow that one to express itself the most, and tell you about itself.

Journal your findings. If you feel inclined, a drawing/sketching/painting exercise can be helpful here. Can you draw/paint each of the characters? Can you turn them into puppets? What do you notice about the way they look?

By naming and personifying our emotions, we allow them an opportunity to emote. When we characterize them, they are no longer entrenched within us, unidentifiable. If the situation allows, return to the issue twenty-four hours after the exercise. Notice if your reaction has changed at all, and how. Remember that the premise of the work is to shift how we relate to our experiences, and in so doing, alter the quality of our lives. Has any more space been created? ■

Practice Allowing the Self

The work of allowing the self is akin to that of avoiding the second arrow. As we explored in Part I, the first arrow is the original pain caused by unavoidable losses, illness, disappointments, rejections; life is full of these. The second arrow is our reactions, and ultimately how we relate to the first arrow. The second arrow is the blame we attach to our situation (whether ourselves or others), running into distractions only to return and feel additional guilt for having done so. While we cannot predict when and how life will fire the first arrows our way, we can work on not shooting ourselves with the second. In other words, we can stop perpetuating our original hurt.

Exercise I: Identifying the Second Arrow

Applied Practice

If we're unaware of our patterns with the second arrow, if we don't know we're firing it, then it's very unlikely we'll take our hands off the bow. For this exercise, commit a day, week, month (or any specified amount of time) to considering the second arrow, and journal your findings. This exercise is quite straightforward. Carry a small journal with you (or note it on a note-taking phone app, for example), and pay attention to the times when something upsetting happens. Then, immediately note:

- What are my bodily reactions?
- Where do I feel it in my body?
- What are the first thoughts/feelings that arise? Self-blame? Blaming another? Guilt? Fear? Sadness?
- What desire comes next? To indulge in sweets? Go shopping? Call someone and complain?

By becoming aware of where our emotional body goes, and where our tendencies reside, we notice the second arrow and create space between us and the tendency to fire it. We learn to abide in the space between reactions, and as a result, the grip of reaction lessens until we no longer feel pulled to react, but rather become capable of not adding another arrow to the first.

You might notice parallels between emotions. If the first arrow makes you angry, the second arrow might be guilt: you feel guilty for being angry. Or the first arrow may be sadness, and the second anger that you're sad. The second arrow requires that we leave the space of the first (often because the second arrow is tied to our experiences of the past and our expectations for the future). The work, then, is to notice and acknowledge the patterns, so we can remain in the present with the first arrow.

Exercise 2: Creative Conversation

Home Practice

Once you've identified one of the second-arrow emotions, explore it further. For this exercise you'll need two pieces of paper (ideally blank with no lines) and two different-colored writing utensils. Place all materials in front of you, and find a comfortable upright seat that allows you to be alert. Begin breathing exercises to come into a relaxed state.

Place one piece of paper and one utensil in front of you on the side of your dominant hand. If you're right-handed, the paper will be in front of you, slightly to the right. Label this piece of paper ME. Place the other piece of paper with the other writing utensil slightly to the side of your nondominant hand. At the top, label the paper with the name of the secondary, reactive emotion you found in Exercise 1 (e.g., SADNESS).

Imagine a conversation with the emotion. This exercise requires a good amount of suspension of judgment, and letting yourself come into your creative mind. You can begin by simply writing a greeting, *Hi, Sadness. How are you?* with your dominant hand on the paper that is labeled ME. Then, respond on the paper labeled with the emotion by writing with your nondominant hand. This will feel extremely slow and cumbersome at first. Notice all of this and keep going. Start a dialogue between the two, and see what develops. Here are a few questions you might consider:

- Why are you here?
- How long have you been around?
- What makes you tick?
- What are you trying to teach me?

There are no wrong questions to ask. Encourage yourself to be fully creative and delve into this often unexplored element, as you express yourself from your non-dominant side. Save the conversation to read at a later time when that same emotion arises. You might be surprised at the responses that emerge when you allow your consciousness to be soft and creative.

Exercise 3: Identifying the Belief

Home Practice

Much of the time, we repeat old patterns because the underlying foundation of how we relate to that area of our lives has not changed, even if the internal circumstances have. Hence, we're caught in the cyclical patterns of, say, dating the same person in different bodies for years, or having the same work issues at every job. Sometimes, we become stuck because our belief structures around those areas are unexplored, unconscious, and based on a premise of separation. This exercise helps us to identify what is happening in these unlit spaces, and sets the stage for transformation.

In the comfort of your personal space, begin as usual by using a breathing technique to calm the body and mind for several minutes. When the lake is relatively still, bring to mind a recurring situation in your life. Say the pattern is that you tend to date people who are emotionally unavailable, or you tend to find work that pays you less than your skill set is worth. Once the situation is identified, notice where in the body you feel it most. Breathe into that space. Pare the problem into a simple, generalized statement and write it on a piece of paper. Then write the word BECAUSE in all capitals For example, you might say, "I date people who are emotionally unavailable BECAUSE _____").

Below, start a list of reasons. Don't think too hard or judge what comes out; just write. This is an exercise in allowing the creative mind to brainstorm without judgment. Once you have a list of reasons, give each reason a score or emotional valency by reading the reasons out loud and seeing which ones create a more visceral physical reaction. Circle the top three. These are your limiting beliefs. Here are couple examples:

- I date emotionally unavailable people because I'm afraid that if someone really gets to know me, they won't actually love me.
- I work for people who don't pay me what I'm worth because I don't think I'm worth that much.

For each limiting belief, identify the underlying core belief:

- I believe I'm not lovable.
- I believe my work isn't worth much.

Now, ask yourself how each belief was useful:

- How has this served me in the past? What have I gotten/am I getting out of this?
- How do I foresee it helping me in the future? What will I get out of this?

For example,

- If I'm not lovable, then someone won't love me and I won't have to love them either.
- If my work isn't worth much, then I won't have to take on more responsibility.

Write and repeat each statement out loud, and see how it feels in the body. Allow that feeling to remain as you notice. By identifying it and allowing it to be there, the relationship changes. Now consider: What would happen if the opposite were true? For example:

- I am lovable: anyone would love to be with me.
- My work is exceptional: any boss would be thrilled with my performance.

Repeat these statements several times, body-scanning and noticing any changes.

Our behavior stems from our thoughts, and many of our thoughts are rooted in belief structures we're unaware of. By paring and identifying these beliefs, we allow them the space to be, so we might clear them. They may not clear initially, but when we realize they're there, they lose power and attachment. When these limiting beliefs no longer linger in the shadows, unnamed and untouched, we recognize them as we engage with others. Slowly, our beliefs are transformed and our behavior changes. ∎

III

PRACTICE THE SHADOW

Carl Jung wisely said, "What you resist not only persists, but will grow in size." Resistance is the opposite of resolution; we cannot resolve anything while we resist it. This is where we begin with the work of allowing. Whereas the proposed exercises on allowing help us discover and explore our barriers to resistance, practicing the shadow digs deeper still, and from a different vantage point. If the lake is a metaphor of our minds, and the reflection is how we see ourselves and the surroundings, then the shadow is the depth and frequency of ripples affecting how we perceive ourselves and others.

We tend to reject what we don't recognize ourselves in—perhaps because on a deeper level we *do* see ourselves in perceived negative traits, and we reject them. This is the basis for blame and judgment, and we explored it in the segment on the Other in Part I. So long as some element of the Other remains alien to us, we resist it. In that alienation is separation, and in separation the experience of wholeness is evanescent at best.

Educator Parker Palmer once said, "Wholeness does not mean perfection: it means embracing brokenness as an integral part of life." We cannot be integrated so long as we don't embrace brokenness within ourselves, others, and the world. Practicing the shadow is precisely the work of yoga: the union of the uncomfortable spaces we often identify outside of ourselves, so we might stop resisting them and, instead, invite them into our wholeness. ■

Exercise I
Identify the Shadow

Home Practice

You'll need a piece of paper and a writing implement. Begin at home within your comfortable, safe space. Engage breathing exercises that help you find a relaxed and alert state. Once you feel clear and ready to begin, bring to mind a person with whom you have a minor difference. As always, when first beginning this work, start with an issue or person that isn't emotionally charged, but rather something/someone causing mild annoyance. Once you have picked your focus, write down five to fifteen traits that bother you about it/them. Try to be specific: "It really irritates me when _____ picks their teeth during a work meeting."

Once you have your traits, read down the list until you find one you feel a medium to strong emotional charge with. Pay attention to the sensations in your body as you read the traits, and notice (and perhaps jot down) where and how you feel it in your body. After you've chosen a trait to work on, hold it in your mind's eye. Ask yourself the following questions:

- What about this trait bothers me?
- Where in my body do I feel discomfort when I contemplate this trait?
- What other people in my life have or have had this trait?
- In what ways do I exhibit this trait myself?
- Under what circumstances does this same trait show up in my own personality?

Once you identify the trait within yourself, choose to express this very trait through creative outlets: it can be a drawing, painting, journaling, or another expression of your choosing.

Recognizing our shadows helps us close the gap between ourselves and the Other. The Other stops being a stranger when we come to admit that we, too, hold these elements within us. ∎

Exercise 2
The Three-Year-Old

Home Practice

Now that you've identified a shadow element (or several), we can work more deeply. Begin, as usual, by creating a comfortable and safe space and employing breathing techniques. When you feel ready, pick one shadow element from the identification exercise above. For this topic, we'll use an example: "I am bothered when my coworker is condescending during meetings." Once the element is picked, ask: *Why is this so important to me?* After you've responded, continue to probe, as a three-year-old might. The discussion might end up looking something like this:

> "I am bothered when my coworker is condescending during meetings."
> *Why is this so important to me?*
> "Because it's good for group morale that everyone treats one another with respect."
> *Why?*
> "Because respect is crucial in work relationships."
> *Why?*
> "Because if someone thinks they're better than everyone else, it creates division."
> *Why?*
> "Because some people are naturally more proficient at certain tasks than others, but ultimately we're all equal."
> *Why is this so important?*
> "Because even if we struggle with tasks, we're all still valuable."
> *Why?*
> "Because effort is what matters most."
> *Why?*
> "Because at some point you will fail, even if you try."
> *Why is that important?*
> "Because there are times I've failed and I'm afraid my efforts won't be taken into consideration."

Once we identify the shadow of our beliefs, the roots of what bothers us, we can ask ourselves where our belief structures came from. Identifying the belief structures breaks the fourth wall (to use the metaphor of the stage from Part I). We're no longer entrenched within the hidden belief; even if we still believe it, we've altered our relationship toward it. ■

Exercise 3
It's Okay to Be "Bad"

Home Practice

Most of us think we're a "good person." We walk through the world trying to be a positive influence or at least attempting not to leave a negative mark. Yet, identifying exclusively with goodness creates a bifurcation within us, and the belief that it's bad to be "bad." Hence, we judge and react against that which we feel is bad. For this exercise, begin in the usual home-practice manner by settling in your space and breathing to create clarity and alertness. Then bring to mind three to five positive qualities you see in yourself. They may be qualities you pride yourself on.

Once you possess your short list, draw a line across from each of the qualities and write the opposite of that quality. For example, if one of your positive traits is "hardworking," then the opposite might be "lazy." If there's emotional valence there, notice it, and pay attention to what it feels like in the body. If you find the thought of being lazy, for example, very bothersome, then this might be an unintegrated shadow. Once you've identified a shadow element, sit with it for a moment. Then, make a list of places in life where it's okay to exhibit that shadow. For example, it might be okay to be lazy on a Sunday afternoon after a long week of work.

Within us, we hold an ocean of opposites, although ultimately they're part of the same whole. When we shun or resist our shadow elements, we perpetuate our internal discomfort because these same hidden elements play a large role in our behavior and in our unconscious reactions. If, instead, we seek to bring light and awareness to these places, then their grip on us releases and our judgments, whether internal or projected, loosen as we gain insight into things as they are.

Identifying and being with our shadow elements closes the gap between self and the Other, until we realize that our many traits are similar. From this place, compassion arises. ■

IV

PRACTICE GREATER MIND

Practicing Greater Mind is about recognizing that our lives and stories are just one thread in a vast quilt of experiences. Think of our metaphor of flying in a plane from Part I: the higher we go, the more we realize how tiny we actually are. When we're in emotional pain and separation, we're fully zoomed in and cannot access the larger expanse of collective experience. All of the exercises we've explored thus far help expand our consciousness and sense of Self, and tap into the Greater Mind, or the unified, non-localized consciousness that is *puruṣa*. The metaphor of the salt from Part I, where we compared the taste of a tablespoon of salt in a cup of water to a tablespoon of salt in a fresh lake, is also an excellent example of Greater Mind. When our container is expanded, the salt (pain, discomfort, suffering) disperses; the water isn't so salty.

As we explored in Part II, these concepts are most useful when they become our practice—something we commit to. As is true with both the first book of the *Yoga Sūtras* as well as with Patañjali's Eight Limbs of Yoga, these practices start with the gross, tangible, and easily accessible and move into subtler spaces. These more nuanced practices come about as happy developments from the foundation laid by the more accessible practices.

Notice, for example, that I seldom use the word *meditation* (or *dhyāna* in Sanskrit), even though many of these exercises might commonly be referred to as "meditations" or "meditation exercises." Classically speaking, meditation is a subtle state that arises, rather than one we make happen. Instead, we're exploring practices in *dhāraṇā*, or concentration.[36] From concentration arises meditation, a more elusive and subtle state. So, whereas we can still speak to practices of Greater Mind and Surrender, the two are ultimately a result of the work done with witnessing, allowing, and shadow work. ∎

Exercise I
Identify Greatness

Home/Applied Practice

It's valuable to identify Greater Mind when we tap into it, though many of us haven't had access to the language or concept, and hence have been unable to name it. By learning to identify Greater Mind, we can study the circumstances that led us to that point, and note important patterns that help dissolve our salt, and open us to the vastness of our lake.

Greater Mind happens when we're pulled out of our individual situation and feel a sensation of openness within our experience. It can feel like an *aha!* moment. Tapping into Greater Mind also has a distinctive feel of a situation loosening it grip. One example that students often bring up in my philosophy seminars is coming into a yoga or meditation class with a particular anxiety or desire (say, whether to buy a pair of jeans they've had their eye on all week) and noticing that after the class those feelings of discomfort and desire are gone, or at least lessened. Usually, the sensation is of one needing less, and feeling more complete.

If this rings a bell, in home practice sit and perform breathing exercises until you're in a place of alert calmness. Then, on a piece of paper, brainstorm circumstances in which you've already experienced Greater Mind. You might notice that as you write, you get more ideas. If the session turns into a free-write, go with it, and see what the mind produces. If you have trouble listing, take a moment to reflect on your childhood or teenage years and ask: *What are some particularly happy memories where I felt like I lost track of time?* Childhood is an easier stage of life (for most, though not all, depending on individual circumstances) to tap into Greater Mind and lose track of time in play, sport, or community, because the ego doesn't fully grip the way it does in adulthood, perhaps because there are fewer experiences to identify with. From this exercise, pick the top three to five places you felt the most tapped into: the most absorbed in process, undefined by story, and expansive. Write them down.

For applied practice, choose a day, week, or month to witness. Pay attention to when you feel internally expansive: where you lose time, fully immersed in your experience. It's likely you'll notice it after the fact, rather than during. Journal what made you feel tapped into Greater Mind, and what sensations you had; or how it felt before, during, and after that experience.

To take the applied practice further, keep a nightly journal of Greater Mind. Each evening, before going to sleep, reflect on the day and find three to five moments of expansion. You may journal about how they felt, what they involved, etc.

By bringing awareness to the effortless moments of Greater Mind that already transpire within our lives, we take ownership of that connection. Then, Greater Mind moves from being an elusive space into one we can learn to re-create as we witness our patterns of connection (and hence our patterns of disconnection, as it's likely that as you journal you'll also shed light on when Greater Mind was zoomed back in to the compressed sense of self). ■

Exercise 2
Beyond-the-Body Scanning

Home Practice

Sit in a comfortable and supported position that allows you to remain alert yet relaxed. Employ breathing exercises. Close or gently soften the eyes and bring all your consciousness and awareness to the center of the body. Imagine you can abide in this space. Take three to five breaths. Then extend outward: bring your awareness to your chest, then your hips. Breathe and stay there. If thoughts arise, acknowledge them, but come back to the breath and the body. Then continue to move from the core to the periphery: bring your awareness to your arms and legs. Breathe into the center of each limb. Imagine that the body is encased in sheaths. Move from organs to bones to muscle tissue to skin, in each area.

Next, move to head, hands, and feet. Scan each. Imagine the anatomy in each, moving outward. Breathe. Notice what you see and what thoughts arise. Then send the awareness to the tips of the body: the fingertips, tips of the toes, crown of the head. Breathe into and send awareness to your outermost edges: imagine they pulse with breath. Next, bring awareness to whatever you're sitting on, that which your bottom is making contact with. Breathe there. Notice the sensations and points of contact and imagine them as an extension of your body. After several breaths, continue to expand outward into whatever those objects are touching, and those objects, and so forth until you've encapsulated the room you're in, the building, the city, state, country, continent. You might zoom out past the planet Earth, past the Milky Way, as far as you'd like to go. Breathe into all of the space you can find.

If on the first try you find it difficult to move beyond the body, don't give up. With practice, concentration will increase from the smallest atom to the greatest of magnitudes.[37] ∎

Exercise 3
Hot-Air Balloon

Home Practice

Identify a situation that feels contracted in your life—one that isn't too emotionally potent. Come to your space and start the breathing exercises. Imagine your situation is like a giant bowling ball. Notice how heavy it is; you might not be able to lift it. Imagine this ball is in your house. How much room does it take up? Now, imagine you're able to take it outside and put it, and yourself, inside the basket of a hot-air balloon. You fire more air into the balloon to leave the ground and rise above your house. The ball might still be quite large relative to your home (which stands for yourself, your inner space). Then fire more hot air and rise still higher. Now you see your immediate neighborhood. Notice how much space the ball takes, how it affects and relates to the immediate circle of things that matter to you. After some breaths and some time exploring the vicinity of your emotional neighborhood, go higher: now you're hovering over your city. How large is the ball compared to your city? How much weight does it have?

   Continue to ascend until you're floating over your city, state, country, or planet. Notice if the bowling ball has gotten any smaller, or at least notice the contrast in size. Then, notice its weight and tension in your body—has it lessened? Journal about your experience. ∎

Exercise 4
Nature

Home Practice: Field Trip

We tend to spend so much time caught in the drama of our lives that we forget we're part of Earth. We are the stuff of forests and seas, mountains and deserts. We are nature. Our ancient ancestors depended immediately and directly on the provisions of Earth in a way that most of us in developed societies are only indirectly connected to. We're often unaffected by droughts or floods that damage crops. We may not know where our food comes from, or the migration patterns of local wildlife. Nonetheless, this disconnectedness from Earth and its patterns can throw us further into our own dramas, and away from the truth that all is cyclical: beginning, ending, and enduring all at once.

Taking our exercises into nature is a beautiful way to connect, firsthand, with Greater Mind. It's a way for us to immerse ourselves and recognize our place in the expanse of creation. This exercise can be completed anywhere in nature: ideally, in a forest or park with lots of vegetation and trees; or at the beach, or in the mountains.

Find a comfortable seat. Locate the breath or employ breathing exercises. Gently open the eyes if they were closed. Look around and find one item: a leaf, an ant, a grain of sand. Look at it, name its attributes. Then zoom out. Notice the area around the leaf: is the leaf on a branch of leaves? Or is it one grain of sand in a section of beach? Is it one wave of the ocean? Stay at this level, and breathe and observe. Zoom out more. What do you see? Are there any repeated patterns? Continue and notice the continual expansion of the object you started with. Notice how you can move your zoom in either direction. You can start with the whole forest and end up with a particle on a leaf on a single tree, for instance. In either direction is an expanding matrix of connectivity. ■

V

PRACTICE SURRENDER

We come, at last, to the subtlest of all the practices, the ninja training of consciousness: surrender. Surrender happens when we finally remove all the sheaths, covers, and blockades we've hidden behind. We give up our need to resist. Surrender is sometimes more easily arrived at after practicing Greater Mind, because there we come face-to-face with the reality of our smallness and the truth that our piece is just one leaf in a vast canopy of experience. We may also touch on the limitation of our perception, in contrast with the greatness we're a part of.

In an attempt to explain human existence in relation to that of the universe, physicist Carl Sagan popularized a cosmic calendar—condensing all time into one year, with one day the equivalent of 40 million years. If the Big Bang is the first second of January 1st, the dinosaurs don't arrive until December 25, and our species doesn't appear until eight minutes to midnight on December 31st. Surrender is realizing we're a blink of an eye in the cosmic calendar. So we let go, completely. ∎

Exercise I
Body-Scanning Hold and Release

Home Practice

Practicing surrender in the body can be a way to deeper levels of surrender. For this exercise, lay on your back on a comfortable surface. Take deep breaths and move the

breath through the body for a few minutes. Notice areas of tension and any entering thoughts. Imagine your breath as a wave washing through your body. Bring your
attention to your toes. Contract them for a round of two breaths, then release. If you
find it helpful, use a mantra like *Let Go* once you release the toes. Move to the calves.
Tighten them, breathe, and release. Repeat the pattern up the body, section by section: thighs, glutes, fingers, forearms, and upper arms, until you end at the head and
face. With each contraction, feel the body tightening and resisting, and with each
release, feel the body letting go completely. Journal what places are more or less difficult to release. ∎

Exercise 2
Help, Please

Home/Applied Practice

Underlying surrender is the belief that we are part of a friendly universe, that things
are going to be okay. Underlying surrender is the faith that we'll bounce back, and the
recognition that we cannot control everything that happens. These may be large pills
to swallow, but asking for help, helps.

Practicing surrender means knowing when to ask for help. This can be true on
a practical level, where you reach out to members of your community or support
system, as well as internally. Asking for help means recognizing that we don't have all
the answers, that our point of view is restricted, and that there's a limit to our abilities.
In asking for help, we're not asking for the situation to change, but for a shift in our
perception and in our relationship to what ails us. In asking for help, we're opening
ourselves up to an alternative point of view, a consciousness that isn't so limited. We're
asking for access to the greater picture, for our hearts to soften to the myriad possibilities outside our realm of consciousness, where boundless creativity, abundance, and
love reside.

Sit in a comfortable place and engage in breathing exercises. Bring to mind
something small you want to surrender to. This can also be done in real time, when
something strikes you and you feel caught within a situation. Imagine yourself
squeezing this situation, as you contracted the muscles in the body-scanning
exercise. Now imagine yourself releasing, as you would muscles. Notice if anything

changes. Then, ask for help: *I see my relationship and attachment to this issue. Please, help me open, release, and surrender.* You can also ask from the perspective of the change having already taken place: *Thank you for helping me expand my mind and my experience with this issue. Thank you, because I have seen another alternative I never thought possible.*

You can use any formulation that resonates with you and comes from within. Notice what happens. The change might be instantaneous, or it might take weeks, months, or even years. The outcome will depend on the quality of the practice, and with practice, the mind and heart will open like a blossoming flower.[38] ∎

Exercise 3
Thank You

Home Practice

We say "thank you" when something has been done for us. We show gratitude after a change in circumstances. In gratitude, we've already let go of a situation. Gratitude can also become a valuable practice that supports the internal work of surrendering. As we've learned, that which we focus on grows in our experience. If we learn to focus on gratitude, then our experience will necessarily change. This exercise on thankfulness has two aspects, and you can practice one or both.

Pick a time of day when you can consistently practice this short exercise. You can choose to devote a small journal to it. Create a comfortable seat and employ breathing exercises to clear the mind. When you're ready, write three to five things that happened in your day that you're grateful for. Write *Thank you for* _____. At the bottom of the page, write one thing you are grateful for that hasn't yet happened, in the same fashion: *Thank you for* _____.

The gratitude journal serves to help us focus on the small (or great) things we have to be thankful for. Even on the worst days, we can name objects of gratitude. This aspect changes our outlook on a perceived issue from resistance to gratitude, as if we've already surrendered it.

As time passes, you might find the gratitude list needs to expand; I encourage you to allow it to do so. The more gratitude we feel, the more surrender we experience. The more surrender we practice, the less resistance arises. The less we resist, the more we allow; the more we love, the more alive we are and the more we show up to meet what really matters: what's here, present, always.

In all of the practices in which we learn to show up, pay attention, and wake up, we practice returning to ourselves at the moment at hand. Presence is the greatest of all homecomings. Even when it's difficult, all of these small daily efforts will one day grace us. This is the promise and gift of yoga. Yoga is there for us when we need it most. As the *Gita* reminds us, on this path effort never goes to waste. ∎

Epilogue

In May 2017, Vannesa and I celebrated Mami's death the way we do every year: we told stories about our parents as we listened to traditional Colombian music, and reminisced about Mami and Papi dancing in our living room back home while filling our bellies with steaming yucca and sweet plantains.

This last celebration, however, was markedly different in two ways. First, it was the twentieth anniversary of Mami's passing. Twenty years. A lifetime by any measure. In that enigmatic quality of memory and time, it seemed as if it was only months ago that I was running my hands through that thick, black mane of hers, and simultaneously that it had been ages since I'd experienced the vibrant warmth of being scooped up in her arms.

Secondly, Vannesa and I were no longer the same as when we held Mami for the last time, on that beautiful afternoon in late May. We were no longer two scared little girls looking into the abyss of orphanhood. On this day, the twentieth anniversary of Mami's death, Vannesa and I had both stepped into another type of mystery that would prove to fundamentally change us both: Motherhood.

Twenty years later, Vannesa and I found home again—not in the tangibility of a physical location, like returning to Colombia or California, or even in a metaphorical sense like finding home in a state of mind. Instead, we'd found our grounding, our family, and ourselves in our sons. We'd come full circle. After delving into death for decades, we'd now gotten to bring about life.

From the moment he was born, my son revealed to me traces of my parents—he has Mami's eyes and silly sense of humor and Papi's intellect and deep inquisitiveness. When I spend time with him, I feel as though I am, in a very real way, spending time with both of my parents. It is truly fascinating, this ubiquitous thing we call family.

In having my son, I came to understand something that no amount of meditation taught me. I came to experience firsthand the love my parents had for me; I came to see Mami from an entirely different vantage point—mother to mother. In this light, her devotion to her daughters has not only become sweeter, but it has become a model for my own parenting. I hope that one day my son feels as loved by me as I do by both of my parents to this day, even in their absence of several decades.

Motherhood has become my primary yoga, and it turns out that my son has brought home the yogic teachings in a way I couldn't anticipate—he makes their relevance palpable. Every day I am met with an important decision: I can choose to mourn the fact that he will never feel Mami's warmth or listen to Papi strum his Brazilian guitar, or I can choose to embody wholeness and love. This is my practice: the daily renewal of a commitment to see and to teach my son what Mami taught me long ago: *Life is worth it.*

Acknowledgments

So many heartfelt thanks are in order. First, to my sister and tiny Buddha, Vannesa, without whom neither I nor this book would be here. This is her story as much as it is mine. Thank you for being there every step of the way, for allowing me to share our journey, and for helping me sculpt it into something manageable. Thanks to those of you who left this realm too soon: my mother, Olga, for being the embodiment of passion, humility, and grace; my father, Jairo, for instilling in me curiosity and nourishing my inquisitiveness; my best friend, James, for seeing me through the darkest of times; and my tia, Myriam, for reading everything I ever wrote. A huge thank you to my midwives during the birthing process of this book: Victoria Moran and Jennifer Vera Faylor—your insights, wisdom, and guidance have been truly invaluable. Thank you to Martin Rowe, whose keen and profound editorial guidance helped me see things I could not see for myself, and for seeing the light in this manuscript.

Thank you to my intellectual teachers for honing my philosophical eye: Eleanor Wittrup, George Randels, Lou Matz, Bob Gregg, and Thomas Sheehan, and special thanks to my graduate advisor, Jean Graybeal, for our work on Heidegger and for melding the mind and the heart. To my teachers on the path: Jhon Tamayo for introducing me to my practice; Kevin Courtney, who with his contagious devotion to this path has helped me cultivate my own; Shanti Kelly for teaching me its embodiment in relation to healing; and the devoted monks and teachers at the Integral Yoga Institute and Ananda Ashram for introducing me to the Sanskrit texts and their classical study.

Thank you to my dearest friend, Suzanne Vyborney, for always believing in me; to Andrew Morrison for his honesty; to Dinis Morais for his support during the editing process; to Dyana Balcazar for her tremendous help so that I could focus on writing; to Ligia Haley for being my cheerleader; to Candace Johnson for her council; to Ron Platzer for his mentorship; to Lillian Eve Moore for her wisdom; Matt Fitzwater for his amazing work on the cover art; to the SD for all its guidance; and to my son Soren, who has deepened, nurtured, and brought home (both figuratively and literally) the magnitude and impact of these teachings in the most beautiful and surprising ways.

Last, but certainly not least, an enormous thank you to all my students who inspired and encouraged me to put my story and my teaching work into book form, and who continue to show up with earnest and curious hearts.

Appendix

Below are the transliteration and translation for key *sūtras* discussed in the text. Translation by its nature is a tricky endeavor: much can be lost without or added through context; and context, particularly of an ancient language, can be difficult to ascertain. For this reason, I've decided to provide three translations for each *sūtra*.

All translations numbered "1" are by the Indologist Edwin F. Bryant in *The Yoga Sūtras of Patañjali: A New Edition, Translation, and Commentary with Insights from the Traditional Commentators* (New York: North Point Press, 2009).

All translations numbered "2" are by Sri Swami Satchidananda, founder of Integral Yoga Institute in New York City, in *Yoga Sūtras of Patanjali* (New York: Integral Yoga Distribution, 2012).

All translations numbered "3" are by B. K. S. Iyengar, founder of the Iyengar system, in *Light on the Yoga Sūtras of Patañjali* (New Delhi: HarperCollins, 2005).

Sūtra I.1 *atha yogānuśāsanam*
1. Now, the teachings of yoga [are presented].
2. Now the exposition of Yoga is being made.
3. With prayers for divine blessings, now begins an exposition of the sacred art of yoga.

Sūtra I.2 *yogaś citta-vṛtti-nirodhaḥ*
1. Yoga is the stilling of the changing states of the mind.
2. The restraint of the modifications of the mind-stuff is Yoga.
3. Yoga is the cessation of movements in the consciousness.

Sūtra I.3 *tadā draṣṭuḥ svarūpe 'vasthānam*

1. When that is accomplished, the seer abides in its own true nature.
2. Then the Seer [Self] abides in His own nature.
3. Then, the seer dwells in his own true splendour.

Sūtra I.4 *vṛtti-sārūpyam itaratra*

1. Otherwise, at other times, [the seer] is absorbed in the changing states [of the mind].
2. At other times [the Self appears to] assume the forms of the mental modifications.
3. At other times, the seer identifies with the fluctuating consciousness.

Sūtra I.5 *vṛttayaḥ pañcatayyaḥ kliṣṭākliṣṭāḥ*

1. There are five kinds of changing states of the mind, and they are either detrimental or nondetrimental [to the practice of yoga].
2. There are five kinds of mental modifications which are either painful or painless.
3. The movements of consciousness are fivefold. They may be cognizable or non-cognizable, painful or non-painful.

Sūtra I.14 *sa tu dīrgha-kāla-nairantarya-stakārāsveito dṛḍha-bhūmiḥ*

1. Practice becomes firmly established when it has been cultivated uninterruptedly and with devotion over a prolonged period of time.
2. Practice becomes firmly grounded when well attended to for a long time, without break and in all earnestness.
3. Long, uninterrupted, alert practice is the firm foundation for restraining the fluctuations.

Sūtra I.15 *dṛṣṭānuśravika-viṣaya-vitṛṣṇasya vaśīkāra-samjñā vairāgyam*

1. Dispassion is the controlled consciousness of one who is without craving for sense objects, whether these are actually perceived, or described [in scripture].
2. The consciousness of self-mastery in one who is free from craving for objects seen or heard about is non-attachment.
3. Renunciation is the practice of detachment from desires.

Sūtra I.16 *tat-paraṁ puruṣa-khyāter guṇa-vaitṛṣṇyam*

1. Higher than renunciation is indifference to the *guṇas* [themselves]. This stems from perception of the *puruṣa*, soul.
2. Where there is non-thirst for even the gunas (constituents of Nature) due to realization of the *Purusha* (true Self), that is supreme non-attachment.
3. The ultimate renunciation is when one transcends the qualities of nature and perceives the soul.

Sūtra I.21 *tīvra-saṁvegānām āsannaḥ*

1. [This state of *samprajñāta*] is near for those who apply themselves intensely.
2. To the keen and intent practitioner this [*samadhi*] comes very quickly.
3. The goal is near for those who are supremely vigorous and intense in practice.

Sūtra I.22 *mṛdu-madhyādhimātratvāt tato' pi viśeṣaḥ*

1. Even among these, there is further differentiation [of this intensity into degrees of] mild, mediocre, and extreme.
2. The time necessary for success further depends on whether the practice is mild, medium, or intense.
3. There are differences between those who are mild, average and keen in their practices.

Sūtra I.30 *vyādhi-styāna-saṁśaya-pramādālasyāvirati-bhrānti-darśanālabdha-bhūmikatvānavasthitatvāni citta-vikṣepās te'ntarāyāḥ*

1. These disturbances are disease, idleness, doubt, carelessness, sloth, lack of detachment, misapprehension, failure to attain base for concentration, and instability. They are distractions for the mind.
2. Disease, dullness, doubt, carelessness, laziness, sensuality, false perception, failure to reach firm ground and slipping from the ground gained—these distractions of the mind-stuff are the obstacles.
3. These obstacles are disease, inertia, doubt, heedlessness, laziness, indiscipline of the senses, erroneous views, lack of perseverance, and backsliding.

Sūtra I.31 *duḥkha-daurmanasyāṅgam-ejayatva-śvāsa-praśvāsā-praśvāsā vikṣepa-saha-bhuvaḥ*

1. Suffering, dejection, trembling, inhalation, and exhalation accompany the distractions.

2. Accompaniments to the mental distractions include distress, despair, trembling of the body, and disturbed breathing.

3. Sorrow, despair, unsteadiness of the body and irregular breathing further distract the *citta*.

Sūtra I.32 *tat-pratiṣedhārtham eka-tattvābhyāsaḥ*

1. Practice [of fixing the mind] on one object [should be performed] in order to eliminate these disturbances.

2. The practice of concentration on a single subject [or the use of one technique] is the best way to prevent the obstacles and their accompaniments.

3. Adherence to single-minded effort prevents these impediments.

Sūtra I.39 *yathābhimata-dhyānād vā*

1. Or [steadiness of the mind is attained] from meditation upon anything of one's inclination.

2. Or by meditating on anything one chooses that is elevating.

3. Or, by meditating on any desired object conducive to steadiness of consciousness.

Sūtra I.40 *paramāṇu-parama-mahattvānto 'sya vaśīkāraḥ*

1. The *yogī's* mastery extends from the smallest particle of matter to the ultimate totality of matter.

2. Gradually, one's mastery in concentration extends from the primal atom to the greatest magnitude.

3. Mastery of contemplation brings the power to extend from the finest particle to the greatest.

Sūtra I.47 *nirvicāra-vaiśāradye' dhyātma-prasādaḥ*

1. Upon attaining the clarity of *nirvicāra-samādhi*, there is lucidity of the inner self.

2. In the purity of nirvicara-samadhi, the supreme Self shines.

3.   From proficiency in *nirvicāra samāpatti* comes purity. *Sattva* or luminosity flows undisturbed, kindling the spiritual light of the self.

Sūtra I.48 *ṛtam-bharā tatra prajñā*
1.   In that state, there is truth-bearing wisdom.
2.   This is rtambhara prajna, or the absolute true consciousness.
3.   When consciousness dwells in wisdom, a truth-bearing state of direct spiritual perception dawns.

Sūtra II.1 *tapaḥ-svādhyāyeśvara-praṇidhānāni kriyā-yogaḥ*
1.   *Kriyā-yoga*, the path of action, consists of self-discipline, study, and dedication to the Lord.
2.   Accepting pain as help for purification, study of spiritual books, and surrender to the Supreme Being constitute Yoga in practice.
3.   Burning zeal in practice, self-study and study of scriptures, and surrender to God are the acts of yoga.

Sūtra II.3 *avidyāsmitā-rāga-dveṣābhiniveśāḥ kleśāḥ*
1.   The impediments [to *samādhi*] are nescience, ego, desire, aversion, and clinging to life.
2.   Ignorance, egoism, attachment, hatred, and clinging to bodily life are the five obstacles.
3.   The five afflictions which disturb the equilibrium of consciousness are: ignorance or lack of wisdom, ego, pride of the ego or the sense of 'I', attachment to pleasure, aversion to pain, fear of death and clinging to life.

Sūtra II.4 *avidyā kṣetram uttareṣām prasupta-tanu-vicchinnodārāṇām*
1.   Ignorance is the breeding ground of the other *kleśās*, whether they are in a dormant, weak, intermittent, or fully activated state.
2.   Ignorance is the field for the others mentioned after it, whether they be dormant, feeble, intercepted, or sustained.
3.   Lack of true knowledge is the source of all pains and sorrows whether dormant, attenuated, interrupted or fully active.

Sūtra II.5 *anityāśuci-duḥkānātmasu nitya-śuci-sukhātma-khyātir avidyā*

1. Ignorance is the notion that takes the self, which is joyful, pure, and eternal, to be the nonself, which is painful, unclean, and temporary.

2. Ignorance is regarding the impermanent as permanent, the impure as pure, the painful as pleasant, and the non-Self as the Self.

3. Mistaking the transient for the permanent, the impure for the pure, pain for pleasure, and that which is not the self for the self: all this is called lack of spiritual knowledge, *avidyā*.

Sūtra II.16 *heyaṁ duḥkham anāgatam*

1. Suffering that has yet to manifest is to be avoided.

2. Pain that has not yet come is avoidable.

3. The pains which are yet to come can be and are to be avoided.

Sūtra II.35 *ahiṁsā-pratiṣṭhāyāṁ tat-sannidhau vaira-tyāgaḥ*

1. In the presence of one who is established in nonviolence, enmity is abandoned.

2. In the presence of one firmly established in non-violence, all hostilities cease.

3. When non-violence in speech, thought and action is established, one's aggressive nature is relinquished and others abandon hostility in one's presence.

Sūtra II.36 *satya-pratiṣṭhāyāṁ kriyā-phalāśrayatvam*

1. When one is established in truthfulness, one ensures the fruition of actions.

2. To one established in truthfulness, actions and their results become subservient.

3. When the sādhaka is firmly established in the practice of truth, his words become so potent that whatever he says comes to realization.

Sūtra II.39 *aparigraha-sthairye janma-kathanatā-sambodhaḥ*

1. When refrainment from covetousness becomes firmly established, knowledge of the whys and wherefores of births manifests.

2. When non-greed is confirmed, a thorough illumination of the how and why of one's birth comes.

3. Knowledge of past and future lives unfolds when one is free from greed for possessions.

Sūtra II.47 *prayantna-śaithilyānanta-samāpattibhyām*

1. [Such posture should be attained] by relaxation of effort and by absorption in the infinite.
2. By lessening the natural tendency for restlessness and by meditating on the infinite, posture is mastered.
3. Perfection in an *āsana* is achieved when the effort to perform it becomes effortless and the infinite being within is reached.

Sūtra II.48 *tato dvandvānabhighātaḥ*

1. From this, one is not afflicted by the dualities of the opposites.
2. Thereafter, one is undisturbed by the dualities.
3. From then on, the *sādhaka* is undisturbed by dualities.

Sūtra III.1 *deśa-bandhaś cittasya dhāraṇā*

1. Concentration is the fixing of the mind in one place.
2. Dharana is the binding of the mind to one place, object or idea.
3. Fixing the consciousness on one point or region is concentration (*dhāraṇā*).

Sūtra III. 2 *tatra pratyayaika-tānatā dhyānam*

1. Meditation is the one-pointedness of the mind on one image.
2. Dhyana is the continuous flow of cognition toward that object.
3. A steady, continuous flow of attention directed toward the same point or region is meditation (*dhyāna*).

Glossary of Sanskrit Terms

āsana	Seat, posture, or stretching pose for the purpose of preparing the body to sit firmly and comfortably for meditation; the third of the eight limbs of *ashtanga yoga*.
ātman	The innermost or highest form of the Self or soul.
avidyā	Ignorance or non-seeing; the mental state of reality that confuses or misidentifies the soul *puruṣa* with the body or other elements of the natural world.
Bhagavad Gītā	"Song of God"; the dialogue between *Arjuna* and *Kṛṣṇa*; a smaller part of the greater work, the *Mahābhārata*.
buddhi	Intelligence, discrimination; the function of judgment and knowledge of the mind.
citta/m	The combined functionings for the three aspects of the mind: *manas* (sense perception), *buddhi* (intelligence), and *ahaṅkāra* (ego); mind-stuff.
dhāraṇā	Concentration; the sixth of the eight limbs of *ashtanga yoga*.
dharma	Duty, nature, or characteristic; that which is specific and distinctive.
dhyāna	Meditation. The absorption into the object of meditation without being disrupted by any thoughts.
duḥkha	Pain, aversion, frustration, suffering.
haṭha yoga	The path of yoga using physical disciplines to stretch the body and direct breath or vital energy. The physical aspect of yoga practice that includes postures, breathing techniques, seals, locks, and cleansing practices.
japa	Repetitive chanting of a *mantra*.

jñāna	Knowledge. *Jñāna Yoga* is the path of yoga that seeks to understand the ultimate truths of reality through discernment between the Self and the non-self.
kleśa	Afflictions, obstacles, obstruction.
manas	The aspect or function of the mind responsible for sense perception.
prakṛti	The material world comprised of movement; nature.
prāṇa	Breathing in the body; vital energy.
puruṣa	Innermost Self, loosely equivalent to the soul, principle of unmoving, non-change.
saṁskāras	The mental imprints, memories, or impressions left in the subconscious mind. Every experience is considered to leave an imprint.
satya	The second yama; truthfulness.
savāsana	Posture in *haṭha yoga* consisting of resting the mind and body; corpse pose.
sūtra	Thread; a philosophical aphorism in which the most information is packed into the fewest words possible.
svādhyāya	The study of scriptures and self-study.
tapaḥ	To burn; distress, or the practice of *tapaḥ*, involving austerity and self-discipline.
viveka	Discriminative discernment; the distinction between *prakṛti* and *puruṣa*, real and unreal.
vrittis	Thoughts, ideas; cognitive act, movement, or modification.

Notes

1. For a thorough history and analysis, see *The Yoga Sūtras of Patañjali: A New Edition, Translation, and Commentary with Insights from the Traditional Commentators* by Edwin F. Bryant (New York: North Point Press, 2009).

2. One of my favorite contemporary titles strictly on the Eight Limbs is *Meditations from the Mat: Daily Reflections on the Path of Yoga* by Rolf Gates and Katrina Kenison (New York: Anchor, 2002).

3. *Sūtra* I.1. As with all references to the *Yoga Sūtras* in these notes, see Appendix for the transliteration and translation.

4. A note on translation: For the sake of clarity and simplicity, I've chosen to stay away from presenting the *Sūtras* in the original Sanskrit in the body of the text, though they can be found in the Appendix, along with transliteration and translations as presented by three different sources.

5. *Sūtras* II.3–4.

6. *Sūtra* II.5.

7. *Sūtra* I.1.

8. *Sūtra* I.3.

9. *Sūtra* I.2.

10. For more in-depth discussion on neuroplasticity, see *The Mind and the Brain: Neuroplasticity and the Power of Mental Force* by Jeffrey Schwartz and Sharon Begley (New York: Regan/HarperCollins, 2003) and *The Brain's Way of Healing: Remarkable Discoveries and Recoveries from the Frontiers of Neuroplasticity* by Norman Doidge (New York: Penguin, 2015).

11. *Sūtra* I.16.

12. *Sūtra* I.15.

13. *Sūtra* I.4.

14. See Kenneth S. Kendler, "Major Depression and Generalized Anxiety Disorder. Same Genes (Partly) Different Environments?" *Archives of General Psychiatry* 49, no. 9 (1992): 716 and Victor Abkevich et al., "Predisposition Locus for Major Depression at Chromosome 12q22-12q23.2," *American Journal of Human Genetics* 73, no. 6: 1271–81.

15. *Sūtra* I.3.

16. *Sūtra* I.4.

17. See Jill Bolte Taylor's *My Stroke of Insight: A Brain Scientist's Personal Journey* (New York: Viking, 2008).

18. I want to be clear that my statements refer to relationships that are *not* abusive or coercive in nature, and that don't place one or more of the people involved in physical, mental, or emotional danger. If you believe that a relationship you're part of is displaying signs of abuse, I encourage you to contact the National Domestic Violence Hotline immediately.

19. *Sūtras* I.21–22.

20. *Sūtras* II.3–5.

21. *Sūtra* II.1.

22. *Sūtras* II.47–48.

23. *Sūtra* II.1.

24. Sri Swami Satchidananda, *Yoga Sūtras of Patanjali* (New York: Integral Yoga Distribution, 2012), 3.

25. Retrieved from R. Wilkins, "Obituary: K. Pattabhi Jois" *Guardian*, June 8, 2009, https://www.theguardian.com/world/2009/jun/08/k-pattabhi-jois-obituary-yoga/

26. *Sūtra* II.39.

27. *Sūtra* II.1.

28. *Sūtra* I.22.

29. *Sūtra* I.40.

30. Brian Walker, *Hua Hu Ching: The Teachings of Lao Tzu* (Livingston, MT: Clark City Press, 1993).

31. *Sūtras* I.30–32.

32. *Sūtra* I.14.

33. *Sūtra* I.39.

34. Anthony de Mello, *One Minute Wisdom* (New York: Doubleday, 1986).

35. *Sūtra* III.2.
36. *Sūtra* III.1
37. *Sūtra* I.40.
38. *Sūtras* I.21–22.

About the Author

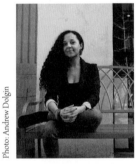

Tatiana Forero Puerta is originally from Bogotá, Colombia. A graduate of Stanford, New York, and Columbia universities, she has taught philosophy and yoga for a decade, including her post as an adjunct faculty member at New York University and the City University of New York. A columnist for *New York Spirit*, *Park Slope Reader*, and *Elephant Journal*, Tatiana is a recipient of the Stanford Garfield Prize in Ethics, the 2017 Pushcart Prize, a 2019 Pushcart Prize Nominee, and a finalist for *Blueshift Journal*'s prize for writers of color. A contributing author of *Religion and Psychology Research Progress*, her work has also appeared in *Able Muse*, *Flock*, *Juked*, *JOY: Journal of Yoga*, and elsewhere. Tatiana lives in New York, where she teaches and writes. You can find out more about Tatiana's work at www.YogaForTheWoundedHeart.com.

About the Publisher

LANTERN BOOKS was founded in 1999 on the principle of living with a greater depth and commitment to the preservation of the natural world. In addition to publishing books on animal advocacy, veganism, religion, and environmentalism, Lantern is dedicated to printing books in the United States on recycled paper and saving resources in day-to-day operations. Lantern is honored to be a recipient of the highest standard in environmentally responsible publishing from the Green Press Initiative.

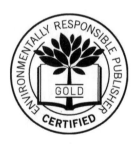

lanternbooks.com

Also by Lantern Books

Tracey Winter Glover
Lotus of the Heart
Living Yoga for Personal Wellness and Global Survival

Ruth Lauer-Manenti
An Offering of Leaves
Foreword by David Life

Ruth Lauer-Manenti
Fell in Her Hands
The Yoga Sutra of Patanjali Translated into Story

Ruth Lauer-Manenti
Sweeping the Dust
Foreword by Sharon Gannon

Mark Whitwell
Yoga of Heart
The Healing Power of Intimate Connection

P100 *like Psalm Poem*